ELEMENTS OF REGIONAL ACCOUNTS

ELEMENTS OF REGIONAL ACCOUNTS

*Papers presented
at the Conference on
Regional Accounts, 1962*

Sponsored by the
COMMITTEE ON REGIONAL ACCOUNTS

Edited by
WERNER Z. HIRSCH

PUBLISHED FOR RESOURCES FOR THE FUTURE, INC.
By The Johns Hopkins Press, Baltimore

© 1964 by The Johns Hopkins Press, Baltimore, Maryland 21218
Printed in the United States of America
Library of Congress Catalog Card Number 64-16309

LIBRARY
FLORIDA STATE UNIVERSITY
TALLAHASSEE, FLORIDA

to the memory of
SELMA GOLDSMITH

COMMITTEE ON REGIONAL ACCOUNTS

WERNER Z. HIRSCH, *University of California, Los Angeles, Chairman*
HAROLD J. BARNETT, *Washington University*
GEORGE H. BORTS, *Brown University*
KARL FOX, *Iowa State College*
DOUGLAS GREENWALD, *McGraw-Hill Publishing Company*
EDGAR M. HOOVER, *University of Pittsburgh*
NATHAN KOFFSKY, *U. S. Department of Agriculture*
CHARLES L. LEVEN, *University of Pittsburgh*
HERMAN MILLER, *U. S. Bureau of the Census*
HARVEY S. PERLOFF, *Committee of Nine, Alliance for Progress; and Resources for the Future, Inc.*
RICHARD RUGGLES, *Yale University*
SIDNEY SONENBLUM, *University of California, Los Angeles*

RESOURCES FOR THE FUTURE, INC.

1755 MASSACHUSETTS AVENUE, N.W., WASHINGTON, D.C. 20036

Board of Directors   REUBEN G. GUSTAVSON, *Chairman,* HORACE M. ALBRIGHT, ERWIN D. CANHAM, THOMAS H. CARROLL, E. J. CONDON (*honorary*), JOSEPH L. FISHER, LUTHER H. FOSTER, HUGH L. KEENLEYSIDE, OTTO H. LIEBERS, LESLIE A. MILLER, FRANK PACE, JR., WILLIAM S. PALEY, LAURANCE S. ROCKEFELLER, STANLEY H. RUTTENBERG, JOHN W. VANDERWILT, P. F. WATZEK

President,   JOSEPH L. FISHER

Vice President,   IRVING K. FOX

Secretary-Treasurer,   JOHN E. HERBERT

    Resources for the Future is a non-profit corporation for research and education in the development, conservation, and use of natural resources. It was established in 1952 with the co-operation of the Ford Foundation and its activities since then have been financed by grants from that Foundation. Part of the work of Resources for the Future is carried out by its resident staff, part supported by grants to universities and other non-profit organizations. Unless otherwise stated, interpretations and conclusions in RFF publications are those of the authors; the organization takes responsibility for the selection of significant subjects for study, the competence of the researchers, and their freedom of inquiry.

    This book is an outcome of one of RFF's regional studies, which are directed by Harvey S. Perloff. The Committee on Regional Accounts, which sponsored the second Conference on Regional Accounts at which the papers contained in this volume were presented, functions under a Resources for the Future grant to the University of California.

RFF publications staff: HENRY JARRETT, *editor;* VERA W. DODDS, *associate editor;* NORA E. ROOTS, *assistant editor.*

CONTENTS

INTRODUCTION, Werner Z. Hirsch xi

FLOWS AND THE ANALYSIS OF REGIONAL
DEVELOPMENT, James M. Henderson 1
COMMENT: George H. Borts 18
Sidney Sonenblum 21

REGIONAL INCOME ACCOUNT
ESTIMATES, Edwin F. Terry 25
COMMENT: Ruth P. Mack 43
Charles E. Ferguson 46

PUBLIC FINANCE AS AN INTEGRAL PART
OF REGIONAL ACCOUNTS, Jesse Burkhead 51
COMMENT: Harvey E. Brazer 77
Karl A. Fox 80

DATA FOR THE PUBLIC-FINANCE
SUB-ACCOUNT, Dick Netzer 87
COMMENT: Lyle C. Fitch 101

AN ACCOUNTS FRAMEWORK FOR METRO-
POLITAN MODELS, Britton Harris 107
COMMENT: Ira S. Lowry 127

THE USE OF INTRAMETROPOLITAN
DATA, William A. Niskanen 131
COMMENT: Lowdon Wingo, Jr. 143

THE MEASUREMENT OF HUMAN
RESOURCES IN A REGIONAL
ACCOUNTING FRAMEWORK, *Leo F. Schnore* . . . 147

COMMENT: *Hal H. Winsborough* 160

MANPOWER MOVEMENTS: A PROPOSED
APPROACH TO MEASUREMENT, *George J. Stolnitz* . . 165

TOWARD AN INTEGRATED SYSTEM OF
REGIONAL ACCOUNTS: STOCKS, FLOWS,
AND THE ANALYSIS OF THE PUBLIC SECTOR,
Harvey S. Perloff and Charles L. Leven 175

COMMENT: *Werner Z. Hirsch* 210

INDEX 215

INTRODUCTION

WERNER Z. HIRSCH
University of California, Los Angeles

During the last few years an intensified effort to develop a system of regional accounts has been proceeding along a number of lines, all closely related. One concern has been the formulation of theories of regional growth and theories of short-run regional interaction. This is not a simple undertaking, and until recently progress has been slow. However, even partial theories of regional growth and short-run interaction are helpful in that they give the accounts builder the specifications essential for his task.

Those working in the field have been aware of the close interdependence between national, regional, and intraregional economic activities, and of the need to develop an integrated set of accounts that can relate all three of these levels. Another key element in these theories of growth and interaction is their general equilibrium character. The interplay between the public and private sectors, between industry and commerce, between places of work and residence, all deserve careful consideration. This complex reciprocal relation must be taken into account to gain a better understanding of the side effects of changed conditions and policies.

It is therefore easily understood that the principal actions of the first Conference on Regional Accounts, held in 1960, were the analysis of the major decision-making problems faced on the subnational level and an attempt to design a set of accounts that would be useful for the examination of alternative solutions to these problems. With the search for comprehensive theories of regional growth and short-run impact continuing, and with design problems retaining the attention of many economists, the second Conference on Regional Accounts aimed at advancing our knowledge by singling out and examining a number of significant parts of regional accounts.

Of the cuts that can be made, some are horizontal and some vertical. Thus, for example, one major concern is to build models that can effectively relate regional economic activity to key aspects of the national economy within an accounts framework. With their aid, short-range and long-range regional changes can be investigated. Likewise, there is need for intraregional models, which can improve our understanding of zoning, land values, and circulation within metropolitan areas.

In addition to this horizontal perspective, a closer look at particular segments of the regional account is warranted. Much emphasis must be placed on the local-government account, because of both strong policy interest and the complexity of the sector. Another key element in a regional account is the household sector. It not only acts as a consumer of goods and services, i.e., is the final buyer for the other sectors, but also furnishes the skills and manpower for their production. It is for the benefit of this sector that the others turn out their goods and services, and thus its importance is paramount.

Finally, a further concern is the separation between flows and stocks in regional accounts. While flows take the form mainly of income and output, stocks emerge as assets or wealth. Although it is desirable to look at stocks and flows separately to gain insight into their behavior, a high order of priority must be given to their effective integration. Thus, the supreme task is to build a well-integrated, three-level flow and stock system comprising national, regional, and intraregional accounts.

A third facet of the building of regional accounts involves their implementation and application to policy determination. In many respects this constitutes the supreme test, and while it must invariably be kept under consideration, a future conference will deal specifically with it.

There is another reason why it is timely to examine carefully key elements of regional accounts. It appears quite clear that because of the complexity of the issues at hand and the large variety of problems facing regions, no single account can be perfected that will be applicable to all regions and to all their problems. A more fruitful approach is to develop a core account accompanied by a number of specialized subsidiary accounts, all of which readily tie in with the first. But what should be the nature of the core and subsidiary accounts? At this moment it appears that some form of regional input-output account can most adequately adapt itself to the functions assigned to a core account. For example, such an account will usually have only a single household column and row and a single local-government column and row. At the same time, however, it will permit the derivation of a very complex household and/or local-government sub-account that can readily be tied into the core account. In addition, it should lend itself to a variety of side calculations in which the interindustry outputs are used as inputs. These side calculations can pertain mainly to regional issues or can be adaptable to an analysis of intraregional questions where the regional input-output account chiefly helps to establish levels of regional economic activity.

These, then, are the relevant approaches that we can take. The Conference emphasized some more than others. For example, long-run regional projections require an enlightened and detailed understanding of a region's economy as part of the over-all posture of the nation, its human and non-human resources, trading opportunities, institutions, preferences. This tie between national and regional economic activity within an accounts framework is the key concern of a paper by James M. Henderson, "Flows and the Analysis of Regional Development." He develops an accounts framework within which the output of a region is related to that of the nation through sets of export multipliers. Fundamentally, a derivative of an open input-output framework is used. The domestic interindustry portion of the matrix has been collapsed and major emphasis is given to trade sub-matrices, charged to give expression to commodity flows between regions. This interregional trading model is likely to prove more useful to short-run impact analysis than to long-run projections and growth analysis, since the trading coefficients are unlikely to be stable. It is being tried out in the Upper Midwest Economic Study, under Henderson's direction, and may be looked upon as an extension of Leon Moses' work on interregional input-output accounts.

The only subnational accounting consistently and readily available for the entire United States on an annual basis is in the income-account estimates prepared by the U. S. Department of Commerce. Work is in progress to extend these efforts to some of the major metropolitan areas. Edwin F. Terry examines the methods used to prepare these accounts. It is quite clear that an effort should be made to extend and improve them further, but at the same time it must be realized that regional income accounts can be expected to shed light on only a select number of regional policy issues, as is so well stated by Ruth P. Mack in her comments on this paper.

Increasing concern in recent years for incidental side effects of public actions, larger scale of public services, and, in general, a desire for improved public decision-making have greatly enhanced the stature of the local-government sector. Regional accounts, it is hoped, should generally expedite the planning of public facilities and long-range fiscal programming. These have been somewhat hampered by the multiplicity of independent government units in most metropolitan areas; but there can be no doubt that in years to come metropolitan areas will see increased cooperation between their balkanized jurisdictions, and some degree of joint policy formulation is likely to result.

As usual, the public sector poses some uniquely intriguing and difficult problems. They range all the way from problems concerned with the establishment of objectives to those of definition and estimation of costs and benefits. Their allocation opens a Pandora's box. Furthermore, there appears to be a need to better relate the activities of the government and quasi-government, i.e., voluntary service organization, sectors. A careful look at some of these issues is taken by Jesse Burkhead, who proposes a government-expenditures account for a region to be classified by function, by level of government, and by form of government organization; distinctions should be made between capital and operating expenditures, and between goods and service and transfer payments. Expenditures so classified could then be arrayed against the clientele population served. Such an account would be a great improvement over existing information systems, although it would appear to fall short of being entirely end-product oriented.

Burkhead introduces an interesting distinction between regional government activities, which are directly affected by the levels of economic activity of households and business firms, and autonomous programs. The first, he points out, exhibit a rather stable and predictable relationship to regional activities and requirements and are mainly circumscribed by the availability of funds. Autonomous government activities, on the other hand, are much more haphazard and virtually impossible to predict.

Dick Netzer considers ways of implementing the public-finance sub-account proposed by Burkhead and carefully investigates the data requirements. His conclusions are rather discouraging, in that he finds that most of the required data are unavailable at present and can be procured only at extremely high cost. He then turns to his recent experience of attempting to develop a 25-year capital budget for the New York metropolitan region. Great gaps in our information system are laid bare, which must be filled before such projections can readily be made. Even capital-expenditure figures for specific facilities in a recent base-year period are seldom available, and what is true for the government sector applies even more stringently to the voluntary-service-organizations sector.

In regions, and particularly in metropolitan areas, much interest centers around land-use, location, and transportation decisions. A number of especially perceptive papers express the hope that these decisions can be better understood and facilitated with the aid of an intraregional-accounts model. Among the most important policy questions, which have already appeared and will continue to develop in metropolitan areas, are those which stem from the differential distribution of activities of urbanites in their capacities as producers and consumers, and the interactions between these distributions. William A. Niskanen takes a critical look at intrametropolitan-decision problems and then places before us a model of the urban space economy. It is an intraregional simulation model in which status variables describe the spatial distribution of activity within an urban area at the beginning of the period under consideration. These variables also constitute the constraints that can be imposed on decisions during the period, and they are joined by input variables which describe the conditions originating outside the metropolitan area, as well as in the public sector. Functional relations describe the changes that appear during the period resulting from the action of the input variables on the status variables. Finally, output variables are used to describe the spatial distribution of activities at the end of the period, thus becoming the status variables at the beginning of the next period. Niskanen hopes that his model not only is useful for organizing data in a consistent manner but also will prove effective as a management tool.

The intrametropolitan space model of Niskanen is akin to that used in the Penn-Jersey Transportation Study. Recently we have witnessed the development of other formal models defining relationships between urban land-use patterns, transportation, and explanatory economic factors. The work of Lowdon Wingo, Jr., the RAND Corporation, and the Northwestern University Transportation Center brings the day near when the requirements of intrametropolitan accounts will be spelled out in great detail.

An initial attempt in this direction has been made by Britton Harris, who explores key problems that must be solved in order to implement Niskanen's and similar models, and their data requirements, within an effective intraregional-accounts framework. Asking what the major variables are that condition the local behavior of decision-makers in metropolitan areas and therefore should be placed into an accounts framework, Harris points to four major groups— the residence of population, the location of economic activities, the channels of movement of people and goods, and land and structures.

He calls attention to the fact that Census data provide much of the required information, except on land use. For this reason he argues that most intrametropolitan-accounts efforts are likely to start with the initiation of major, sophisticated, *ad hoc* local planning or transportation studies requiring detailed land-use information. The accounts should be set up so that they can readily be integrated with available Census data and can themselves easily be updated, to produce time-series information.

Since most regional economic activity is carried out by people for their common benefit, it is of little surprise that regional accounts pay major attention to what is often referred to as the household, human resources, or the human-capital sector. The exceptionally rapid evolutionary changes that have occurred in recent years as by-products of urbanization, mechanization, and automation have impinged on the individual's liberty of choice, privacy, health, and preferences, as well as on group behavior. These forces have affected both the geographic and the vertical mobility of Americans. The "advance guard" in our cities lives a distinctly different life from that of the rest of the population, particularly the recent newcomers. But the transfer of tastes is speedy, as is apparent in the inevitable appearance of some facsimile of exclusive and expensive articles on dime-store counters.

Leo F. Schnore considers some of these issues. Mindful of social and spatial mobility, he is concerned with interactions among people who engage in a variety of transactions. People constitute a stock of human resources at a point of time; the stock undergoes far-reaching changes as the clock ticks away. Schnore attacks the

Introduction

problem of designating a useful areal unit, pointing to the host of alternative objectives which prevent an easy accord. Candidates for such a unit proposed by various scholars vary all the way from the trinity of persons, parcels, and street sections to city blocks, census tracts, counties, and, finally, Standard Metropolitan Statistical Areas.

Placing multidimensional mobility of human resources into a regional-accounts framework is the task that George J. Stolnitz sets for himself. He proposes an ingenious scheme to analyze the impact of a variety of forces on the locational and occupational moves of people. He proposes the development of a two-dimensional manpower "from-to" table. The dimensions would be the industrial or occupational status of the worker and the geographic region. Such a matrix would contain information about the movements of the labor force among industrial or occupational and regional classes during a given period. It would make possible a better understanding of the history of the regional, industrial, and occupational characteristics of a labor force currently engaged in a specified industry and location.

The prospects of such a matrix are exciting, and it appears that much of the information can come from existing Census data. While registration systems such as those in existence today in Sweden offer a very rich source of information, useful for the construction of such a matrix, and are attractive to such human ecologists as Schnore and Hal H. Winsborough, they do not appear necessary. Furthermore they are repulsive to many Americans and are unlikely to be instituted in the United States in the near future.

Virtually all urban-government decisions are directed toward people and property. People own stocks of property and earn flows of income. Taxes are related to these stocks and flows, as are government service requirements. Thus, while it is mandatory that regional accounts incorporate stocks as well as flows, and integrate them, such an effort is most difficult. Harvey S. Perloff and Charles L. Leven attempt to relate stocks and flows within a regional-accounts system with special reference to the government sector. The system that is developed not only is designed to record historical changes in the quantity and quality of resources but also attempts to specify relations between stocks and levels and composition of resource flows. The emphasis rests on an asset inventory and on flow-stock and stock-flow analyses.

It is hoped that an integrated stock-flow account will facilitate our understanding of regional growth. With the aid of comparable information for different regions at different points in time, various suggestive hypotheses could be tested, all bringing the day nearer when we will have a more general regional-growth theory. Thus the Perloff-Leven paper makes a major contribution not only in tying stock and flows together but in relating both to the local-government and human-resources sectors.

However, because of the complexity of the task and the relatively early stage of development in which regional-accounts work now stands, decision-makers would be mistaken to expect regional accounts to perform wonders. Their great attraction is that they provide a consistent methodology for the organization of information-flow systems to facilitate private and public decision-making. They permit simulation of alternative conditions and an understanding of their relative impact on the region in the light of clearly defined criteria. The day is approaching when a major applied effort on a pilot basis can be started to put our present knowledge to test and, hopefully, to work.

FLOWS AND THE ANALYSIS OF REGIONAL DEVELOPMENT

JAMES M. HENDERSON

University of Minnesota

Figures are not available, but the increase in regional research in terms of dollars spent and scholars engaged has been enormous during the past decade. The existence of depressed, distressed, and disorganized areas even in times of general prosperity has become increasingly evident to the public in general and the foundations in particular. More and more local groups have striven to obtain economic studies of their particular areas. A number have succeeded.

Research growth has resulted in an increased demand for regional data. Those who presented papers at the Conference on Regional Accounts were endeavoring to increase the data supply either directly or indirectly. Following the precept of Adam Smith, the chairman of the Conference assigned different aspects of regional accounts to the various participants. Flow accounts were the assignment for this participant.

The assignment has been taken quite literally. The accounts stressed here center upon flows, i.e., interregional movements, of goods and services and, to a lesser degree, people. Such information is considered fundamental for analyses of relations among national economies, but it is usually ignored in analyses of relations among regional economies. This differential approach is discussed briefly in Section 1.

A system of accounts centering upon interregional flows is presented in terms of definitional equations in Section 2. The accounts cover employment, income, and population in addition to flows. They offer promise of implementation on a comprehensive basis for some reasonably detailed regional classification. States and major Standard Metropolitan Statistical Areas (SMSA's) probably provide a minimum necessary regional breakdown.

The accounts become useful for the analysis of regional development once they are available for two or more enumeration periods. Regional development over time then can be analyzed in terms of changes in the values of the account variables and their associated parameters.

The account framework is designed with a view toward generality in order to serve a variety of purposes and types of analysis. At the same time it is purposefully kept simple. There are many types of information that the author wishes were available or easily attainable that are not included within the basic framework. The framework is certainly open-ended.

A few of many possible uses of the accounts for regional comparison, projection, and explanation are suggested in Sections 3 through 5 respectively.

1. THE REGION-NATION APPROACH

The predominant regional research mode involves the study of a particular region as contrasted with the United States as a whole. A region's specialization is characterized in terms of its shares of national activities, and typically regional projections are derived from national projections.

The predominance of the region-nation approach is the result of several factors: (1) interest is usually confined to a single region;[1] (2) most data available on the regional level are also available as national aggregates; and (3) the nation as a whole provides a

---

[1] The region-nation approach is also used in cases of interregional analysis. Here the region-nation approach is applied for many regions and the individual results are contrasted. See Harvey S. Perloff, Edgar S. Dunn, Jr., Eric E. Lampard, and Richard F. Muth, *Regions, Resources, and Economic Growth* (Baltimore: The Johns Hopkins Press, 1960).

convenient and meaningful standard for comparison. The region-nation approach tells little about the process of specialization and trade, but it is workable and provides answers for some important questions.

The wide use of the region-nation approach with its small emphasis upon interregional trade has led to an almost complete divorce of regional analysis from international-trade analysis despite the similarity of the basic process under analysis. A large body of international-trade theory provides little aid for regional analysis.[2] This is something of a paradox since interregional trade conforms more closely to the classic assumptions of international-trade theory than does international trade. Trade among regions takes place without the barriers associated with national boundaries. Once a focus is placed upon interregional trade and data are gathered covering the volume and directions of such trade, regional theory will be in a position to benefit from accumulated international trade theory.

2. A SYSTEM OF FLOW-ORIENTED ACCOUNTS

Method. Regional accounts are presented in terms of definitional equations for past years. These identities are similar to the relations that describe national-income, input-output, and money-flows accounts. When the framework is extended for analysis, the equations provide building blocks and some of the account variables will become variables in a mathematical sense.

In the notational scheme used below, upper-case letters designate account variables; lower-case letters designate parameters, rates, and ratios. Each account variable is defined for a particular year. Superscripts denote regions and subscripts denote sectors.

It is assumed that the United States contains s regions. These may be states, SMSA's or some other geographic classification. Economic activities are partitioned into n sectors which encompass all employment including government.

[2] There are exceptions, of course. See, for example, Leon N. Moses, "A General Equilibrium Model of Production, Interregional Trade, and Location of Industry," *Review of Economics and Statistics*, 41 (Nov. 1960), 373–97.

Trade, Output, and Use. Interregional trade levels are defined for each sector for each pair of regions. The account variable A^{hk}_j denotes the quantity of the gross output of sector j which was produced in region h and used in region k during the year for which the accounts are defined. These flows cover services as well as goods.

Use is defined very broadly. It is total demand including interindustry receipts, final demand by consumers, and inventory accumulation. Trade, output, and use levels are measured in gross terms in relation to value-added measures. Practical considerations generally require that constant-dollar values serve as the units of measurement. The units visualized here are close to the Census of Manufactures "value of shipments" with corresponding measures for non-manufacturing sectors, e.g., the definitions utilized for input-output analysis. The double counting in income terms which is involved in using these units is essential for regional analysis. Each output must be measured whenever it is eligible for interregional movement.

The gross output of sector j in region h, X^h_j, equals the sum of all outflows from j:

$$(1) \qquad X^h_j = \sum_{k=1}^{s+1} A^{hk}_j \qquad (h=1, \ldots, s), (j=1, \ldots, n)$$

where X^h_j is the gross output of sector j in region h. Region $(s+1)$ represents the world outside the United States; $A^{h,\,s+1}_j$ is the level of foreign exports of j from h. Equation 1 includes A^{hh}_j, the amount of j produced and used within region h, and therefore exhausts the total output of h.

The amount of j used in k, U^k_j, equals the sum of all inflows to k:

$$(2) \qquad U^k_j = \sum_{h=1}^{s+1} A^{hk}_j \qquad (k=1, \ldots, s), (j=1, \ldots, n).$$

As before, A^{kk}_j is included. Here the $A^{s+1,\,k}_j$ are imports from foreign countries.

A region's output and use differ by the amount of its net trade. On the national level net trade is often small in relation to total output and it is often not necessary to distinguish output and use. On the regional level output and use are often quite different, and their distinction is essential.

Relations 1 and 2 can be presented in convenient tabular form for each sector. Table 1 contains hypothetical numbers for sector j and emphasizes the double-entry nature of trade accounts. The flow A^{hk}_j is contained in the hth row and k^{th} column of Table 1. For example, the flow from region 2 to region 3 is 5. Gross-output levels are given by row totals and use levels by column totals. Row 4 contains imports from foreign countries, and column 4 contains exports to foreign countries. The system balances in that national output plus foreign imports equals national use plus foreign exports.

TABLE 1. Output, Trade, and Use Levels for Sector j

From \ To	1	2	3	4	Output
1	300	70	30	100	500
2	10	50	5	35	100
3	—	—	20	5	25
4	40	25	10	—	75
Use	350	145	65	140	700

Several observed characteristics of trade-level information are suggested by the figures in Table 1. Apparent cross-hauling exists, i.e., the output of sector j moves both from region 1 to region 2 and from 2 to 1. Classic trade theory precludes cross-hauling. It will, however, exist in any data that can be collected. Cross-hauling may result from the aggregation of individual goods to form a sector. It may result from the definition of regions as areas rather than points. Finally, it may represent inefficient distribution.

Region 1 is a net exporter of j, i.e., its output exceeds its use. The other three regions are net importers. The country as a whole is a net exporter since exports (140) exceed imports (75).

The estimation of trade-level information of the type outlined in Table 1 is a major data-collection task. It is not, however, insurmountable. Trade levels for non-service industries have been estimated on a limited basis for the Upper Midwest Economic Study.[3]

If output levels are measured in value terms, the trade data will

---

[3] See Bruce F. Duncombe, *Upper Midwest Commodity Flows, 1958*, Upper Midwest Economic Study, Technical Paper No. 4 (Oct. 1962).

yield regional balances of payments for goods and services as a by-product:

$$(3) \quad B^h = \sum_{j=1}^{n} X_j^h - \sum_{j=1}^{n} U_j^h \quad (h=1,\ldots,s)$$

where a positive B^h signifies a mercantilistic favorable balance of trade, and a negative value signifies an unfavorable balance. Such balance-of-trade figures omit capital flows and a number of invisible items, but nevertheless would be quite valuable.

Employment. Employment levels by sector and region, denoted by E_j^h, are account variables of major importance for regional as well as national analysis. Regional employment variables require little discussion because of their wide current use. At the moment complete regional employment data do not exist, but such data could be derived from information collected by the state Departments of Employment Security without a major new data-collection effort.[4]

Income. The distinction between income produced and income received is important on the regional level. Income-received data, i.e., personal-income data, have been available on the state level for some time. Income-produced data are more difficult to obtain but hopefully will be more readily available in the future.[5] Again the task is difficult but not insurmountable.

Income produced in region h, Y^h, is defined as the income payments to labor, W_j^h, and other factors of production, V_j^h, by all sectors plus a residual item, R^h:[6]

$$(4) \quad Y^h = \sum_{j=1}^{n} W_j^h + \sum_{j=1}^{n} V_j^h + R^h \quad (h=1,\ldots,s).$$

[4] Employment Security data appear preferable to Census data because of wider coverage. See R. Stephen Rodd and James M. Henderson, *Employment and Earnings in the Upper Midwest: 1950–1960*, Upper Midwest Economic Study, Study Paper No. 5 (Dec. 1962).

[5] See George H. Borts, "The Estimation of Produced Income by State and Region," in National Bureau of Economic Research, Studies in Income and Wealth (forthcoming volume).

[6] The residual item equals the sum of undistributed profits, contributions for social insurance, corporate-profits tax, and the excess of wage accruals over disbursements.

A transition to regional personal income is achieved by replacing the residual item by a term equal to the difference between the income earned in other regions and paid to persons resident in h and income earned in h and paid to persons resident in other regions.

Population and Migration. Regional population figures are available in great detail for Census years, and intercensal estimates are usually available. The interregional-flow picture would be nearly complete if gross migration data were available giving the residential movements of people between each pair of regions during a specified time period. These data would provide a basis for the analysis of labor movements parallel with that for the analysis of goods-and-services movements. Unfortunately such gross migration data are not available and there is little prospect that they will be available in the near future. Hopefully, the 1970 Census of Population will be designed to move further in the direction of gross migration data.

Two alternatives to complete gross migration data are currently available. Each will allow a limited introduction of migration into regional analyses. The 1960 Census of Population provides information on gross in-migration from a limited number of origins. People who moved between 1955 and 1960 were classified as to whether their previous residence was (1) same county, same state; (2) different county, same state; (3) different state; (4) abroad; or (5) unknown.

Net migration by region has been estimated from differently dated population data with the use of indirect methods.[7] The net migration of people to or from region h during a period is defined residually as the actual change of population during the period less natural population growth, i.e., excess of births over deaths, implied by the initial population. A positive difference indicates net in-migration and a negative figure indicates net out-migration.

---

[7] See Larry A. Sjaastad, *Migration and Population Growth in the Upper Midwest: 1930–1960*, Upper Midwest Economic Study, Study Paper No. 4 (July 1962); and U.S. Bureau of the Census, *Components of Population Change, 1950 to 1960, for Counties, Standard Metropolitan Statistical Areas, State Economic Areas, and Economic Subregions,* Current Population Reports, Series P–23, No. 7 (Nov. 1962).

The net migration estimates are comparable to net balance-of-payments estimates. They provide no information regarding total in- and out-migration, or flows.

3. DERIVED PARAMETERS

A number of parameters of interest may be derived from the accounts outlined in the last section. These can provide bases for comparisons among regions that are not dominated by region size. More important, they can provide central elements for regional analyses.

Trade Coefficients. Trade coefficients are defined with respect to the source of supply of each output used in each region:

(5) $\quad a_j^{hk} = A_j^{hk} / U_j^k \quad (h, k = 1, \ldots, s+1), (j = 1, \ldots, n)$.

By the definition of equation 2 the sum of these coefficients over all supply sources, i.e., over h for fixed k and j, equals unity.

The trade coefficients summarize rather complex trade relations among regions. Their use allows a consideration of the specific regional markets supplied by each region; without them we are limited to the common assumption that all regions produce for an amorphous national market. An early study of railroad information showed a marked stability of trade coefficients over time.[8] Trading patterns appear to change slowly. If such stability is demonstrated by the trade coefficients described here, the analytical implications are enormous. Past data can form a reasonable basis for the analysis of future periods.

If trade coefficients do not prove stable, information covering their values over time is even more important, since it will provide the wherewithal to investigate the nature of their change.

Empirical estimates of trade coefficients for the Upper Midwest region reveal general declines in values as distance from purchasing region increases.[9] This suggests that transmission effects from a

[8] Leon N. Moses, "Interregional Input-Output Analysis," *American Economic Review*, 45 (Dec. 1955), 803–32.
[9] See Duncombe, *op. cit.*

region's neighbors may be quite important for an explanation of its growth. A region near California, with a relatively high demand for its products by California, may receive a much greater growth stimulus than would be suggested by an analysis of its share of national output.

Trade coefficients also provide information about the effects of specialization and comparative advantage. If region h supplies commodity j to region k in excess of the amount one would expect on the basis of size, h obviously has some advantage in k's market.

Productivity Coefficients. These coefficients are simply output-labor ratios:

$$(6) \qquad x_j^h = X_j^h / E_j^h \qquad (h = 1, \ldots, s), (j = 1, \ldots, n).$$

The productivity coefficients will prove useful for future projections and provide further information for analyses of regional advantage. They provide the important linkage between demand and employment. At present no one knows the nature, extent, or magnitude of regional-productivity variations.

Income Coefficients. These provide a linkage between income and employment:

$$(7) \qquad w_j^h = W_j^h / E_j^h \qquad (h = 1, \ldots, s), (j = 1, \ldots, n).$$
$$(8) \qquad v_j^h = V_j^h / E_j^h \qquad (h = 1, \ldots, s), (j = 1, \ldots, n).$$

They also provide a basis for a comparison of regional-income levels. It would be of particular interest to compare differentials in regional-income coefficients with differentials in regional-productivity coefficients. The quotient w_j^h / x_j^h is the share of sales revenue paid to labor.

Demand Coefficients. These coefficients relate income produced and use:

$$(9) \qquad b_j^k = U_j^k / Y^k \qquad (k = 1, \ldots, s).$$

They are the least revealing of the coefficients because of the relative paucity of information on the demand as contrasted with the supply side. The analysis of the demand side can be greatly extended in those few instances where regional input-output tables are available.

Growth Rates. Growth analysis may begin once accounts are available for two or more enumeration years. A variety of growth measures may be derived from the accounts. Growth rates, positive or negative, may be calculated for each of the variables and parameters by the division of first differences by initial values. The growth rates will often serve as the key variables in analyses of regional change.

A Missing Link. High correlations and significant regression coefficients can be obtained by the use of regional population change to "explain" regional employment change, or by the use of employment change to "explain" population change. Such correlations, however, are rather spurious. Population and employment are the same once adjustments for participation and unemployment are made. A linkage between the two is necessary. Analysis may then proceed to explain one and the other will follow from the linkage. The parameters thus far described can be computed directly from the accounts of Section 2. A useful linkage between population and employment is not so easily obtained.

One simple linkage is provided by aggregate population-support coefficients. It is assumed that each job in region h provides support for p^h persons. Total population in h then equals employment in h multiplied by p^h, plus the unemployed and their dependents, plus the number of persons who live in h but are neither labor-force members nor their dependents. We can estimate these coefficients by subtracting estimates of the last two categories from h region's total population and dividing the residual by its total employment.

There may be merit in a sector disaggregation of support coefficients. Differences apparently exist. For example, a job in a sector with a high female participation can normally be expected to support a smaller number of persons than a job in a sector with a lower female participation. Furthermore, differential income levels among sectors may affect support coefficients.[10] The "proper" method for a definition of support coefficients is an open question. However, some linkage is essential for a complete analysis of regional development.

4. COMPARISON

Methods. A great deal of current regional analysis involves historical comparisons between regions or between individual regions and the United States as a whole. The body of data described in Sections 3 and 4 can serve as raw materials for a wide variety of such analyses.

A number of simple comparisons of growth and structure are immediately obvious. Employment, population, per-capita-income and other growth rates for each region can be contrasted with corresponding rates for the nation and other regions.

The accounts are easily adaptable for the proportionality-differential shift analyses currently popular in regional economics.[11] An analysis akin to these, but with emphasis upon the flow coefficients and regional markets, is presented as an illustration of the use of the current system of accounts for comparative study.

A Market Comparison. A region may receive a stimulus because of rapid growth of its major external markets, usually near-by markets. Similarly, a slow growth of its external markets can dampen its growth.

From equations 1, 5, and 6, the total employment in h during year t directly attributable to demands in external regions, $\bar{E}^h(t)$, can be expressed as

$$(10) \quad \bar{E}^h(t) = \sum_{j=1}^{n} \frac{1}{x_j^h(t)} \left[\sum_{\substack{k=1 \\ k \neq h}}^{s} a_j^{hk}(t)\, U_j^k(t) \right] \quad (h = 1, \ldots, s)$$

where a time script is added to the variables and parameters. If the bracketed term for $k = h$, i.e., the employment attributable to

---

[10] One might allow support coefficients to vary with regard to sex or income level rather than sector.
[11] See Perloff, Dunn, Lampard, and Muth, *op. cit.*, pp. 70–74 *passim*.

what h supplies itself, were included, the right-hand side of the above equation would equal total employment in h.

Market share and size both influence the growth of a region's external demand. The flow coefficients a_j^{hk} give h's share of its external markets. If these coefficients increased rapidly enough, h's external demand would experience above-average growth even though use levels in its external markets grew at below-average rates. Similarly, declines in h's market shares can offset above-average growth in its external markets. The influence of size is reflected in the growth of use levels in h's external markets. Rapidly growing markets can provide a major growth stimulus even though a region's market shares are declining.

The growth rate for h's external demand from year t to year $(t+\alpha)$ can be separated into components which reflect the influences of market share and size:

(11)
$$\mu^h(t, t+\alpha) = \frac{\bar{E}^h(t+\alpha) - \bar{E}^h(t)}{\bar{E}^h(t)} = d^h(t, t+\alpha) + e^h(t, t+\alpha)$$
$$(h = 1, \ldots, s)$$

where

(12)
$$d^h(t, t+\alpha) = \frac{1}{\bar{E}^h(t)} \sum_{j=1}^{n} \sum_{k=1}^{s+1} \left[\frac{a_j^{hk}(t+\alpha)}{x_j^h(t+\alpha)} - \frac{a_j^{hk}(t)}{x_j^h(t)} \right] U_j^k(t)$$

and

(13)
$$e^h(t, t+\alpha) = \frac{1}{\bar{E}^h(t)} \sum_{j=1}^{n} \sum_{k=1}^{s+1} \left[\frac{U_j^k(t+\alpha)}{x_j^h(t+\alpha)} - \frac{U_j^k(t)}{x_j^h(t)} \right] a_j^{hk}(t+\alpha).$$

The market-share component (12) gives the external-demand growth rate which would have been realized if external-use levels had remained unchanged. The size component (13) gives the rate which would have been realized if use levels exhibited realized change and market shares were at their terminal values.

5. PROJECTION

Data and Method. Projections of the values of regional variables into the future is a major task of most regional studies. The art of regional projections as now practiced is in need of considerable refinement. Better data are an obvious first step. The account system presented here should aid in this regard.

The art of regional projection is also in need of methodological refinement. If adequate explanatory equations for key regional variables were available, a much refined projection methodology could be developed. However, such equations are currently in short supply. A number of refinements are nevertheless possible, and the account framework of Section 2 should prove helpful.

The accounts describe regional structures in terms of a system of simultaneous equations. This system is definitionally true for an enumeration year. It is also definitionally true for any future year for which projections are desired. The system contains more variables and parameters than equations. If there are m equations, these generally can be solved for m of the account variables in terms of the remaining variables and parameters.[12] These m variables are classed then as endogenous, i.e., their future values are determined once values are projected for the remaining parameters and variables. Such a system provides consistent results, a feat not always achieved by current methods. In addition it provides a means for convenient checks. One can independently estimate some of the endogenous variables and compare the estimates with estimates for the same variables derived from the equation system. If corresponding values differ by more than a "tolerable" level, projection methods need reappraisal.

The account equations can be solved for many different sets of endogenous variables. The selection of a specific set will depend upon specific projection objectives and the particular data which are available. An illustrative system similar to that being used for the Upper Midwest Economic Study is briefly described.

[12] There are exceptions to this rule.

An Illustrative System. The United States and foreign trade are represented by thirteen regions. The regions numbered 1 through 6 are the six Upper Midwest states in which interest is centered. The remaining seven are external. Output, use, employment, and income for the Upper Midwest states are selected as endogenous variables. Parameters for the Upper Midwest states and external-use levels are the exogenous quantities to be projected.

The properties of the system may be illustrated through consideration of the endogenous income-produced levels. From equations 4, 6, 7, and 8 levels of income produced in the Upper Midwest are:

$$Y^h = \sum_{j=1}^{n} \beta_j^h X_j^h + R^h \qquad (h = 1, \ldots, 6)$$

where $\beta_j^h = (w_j^h + v_j^h)/x_j^h$ is the proportion of sales revenue paid to factors.

Substituting from equations 1, 5, and 9,

(14) $$Y^h = \sum_{j=1}^{n} \beta_j^h \sum_{k=1}^{6} a_j^{hk} b_j^k Y^k + \sum_{j=1}^{n} \beta_j \sum_{k=7}^{13} a_j^{hk} U_j^k + R^h$$
$$(h = 1, \ldots, 6).$$

The six equations of 14 are expressed in a matrix notation as

(15) $$Y = \sum_{j=1}^{n} \beta_j a_j b_j Y + \sum_{j=1}^{n} \beta_j a_j^{\circ} U_j + R$$

where Y and R are six-component column vectors of income produced and residual income levels respectively, β_j and b_j are 6×6 diagonal coefficient matrices, a_j is a 6×6 trade coefficient matrix describing trade within the Upper Midwest, a_j° is a 6×7 matrix covering trade from Upper Midwest locations to external regions, and U_j is a seven-component vector of use levels in external regions.

Solving equation 15 for Y,

(16) $$Y = [I - \sum_{j=1}^{n} \beta_j a_j b_j]^{-1} [\sum_{j=1}^{n} \beta_j a_j^{\circ} U_j + R]$$

Upper Midwest income levels are thus expressed in terms of Upper Midwest parameters, residual-income levels, and external-use levels. Equation 16 is definitionally true for any enumeration year t. The projection of Upper Midwest income levels for a future year requires the estimation of the parameters and external variables on the right-hand side of 16. Once these are projected, income follows. Furthermore, Upper Midwest employment, output, and use levels follow from the income projections by a simple substitution in the appropriate account equations.

The parameters and exogenous variables on the right-hand side of equation 16 are being estimated by a variety of methods. Some parameters are assumed to remain unchanged, some are modified by *ad hoc* methods, and some are estimated from behavior equations. The exogenous variables are derived mainly from the National Planning Association's regional projections.

Effects of parametric variation are easily calculated from equation 16 once a basic set of projections has been made. It is only necessary to insert alternative values for one or more parameters and/or exogenous variables to calculate changed income values.

Modifications. The Upper Midwest framework is provided merely as an illustration of a general method. Other applications may require modifications of the framework as to the specification of parameters and endogenous and exogenous variables.

6. EXPLANATION

Projection vs. Explanation. Projection involves the estimation of future values for some variables and/or parameters. Explanation involves a determination of the values of one or more of the variables or parameters within the framework of a behavioral model formed by an equation or system of equations. The dividing line between the two is not always distinct. The projection framework presented in the last section, for example, can be converted into an explanatory model by the addition of behavior assumptions.

Correlation and Regression Analyses. These methods are widely used in economics and can be used to advantage for regional applications if the body of information represented by the account variables is available. These methods measure degrees of linear association among variables and/or parameters. We know very little of significance about association among regional variables, and some fairly simple regressions can provide information which is both of interest in itself and helpful for the construction of more complex models.

It is perhaps worth while to insert a word of caution at this point. It is not difficult to find high correlations that are of little interest between regional variables. On a cross-sectional basis migration rates and employment-growth rates exhibit a high positive correlation. This is not surprising, since they are close to being the same thing.

Size can result in largely spurious correlations. Generally, the values of variables are large in a large region and small in a small region. As a result, relatively "good" regression results can be obtained from a cross-sectional analysis without size adjustment. A switch to ratios independent of size usually results in much lower R^2 values.[13] Such problems may never disappear, but better information will greatly widen the horizen for experimentation.

A Few Hypotheses. Many statements, assertions, and suspicions can be stated as statistical hypotheses and subjected to test in terms of simple or multiple regression equations. A few examples in terms of simple regression equations are provided here:

I. Regional growth is dominated by the industry mix toward or away from rapid-national-growth industries:

$$r^h(t) = \xi + \eta \lambda^{h\circ}(t)$$

where ξ and η are regression coefficients and $\lambda^{h\circ}$ is the sum of the industry weights for h for those industries with above-average national-growth rates. The hypothesis will be rejected unless η is positive and significant.

II. Changes in wage-rate differentials from the national average within a given sector are increased by rapid growth and decreased by slow growth as a result of labor-supply pressures:

$$[w_j^h(t+\alpha) - w_j(t+\alpha)] - [w_j^h(t) - w_j(t)] = \xi + \eta r_j^h.$$

[13] This problem was encountered by W. R. Thompson and J. M. Mattila; see their *An Econometric Model of Postwar State Industrial Development* (Detroit: Wayne State University Press, 1959).

A regional cross section for industry j provides data for the test of this hypothesis. Here again η must be positive and significant to avoid rejection.

III. People move in response to income differentials, i.e., migration rates, m^h, are directly related to income differentials:

$$m^h(t, t+\alpha) = \xi + \eta[w^h(t) - w(t)].$$

Here η must be positive and significant.

IV. Current employment-growth rates, r^h, can be explained by past growth rates:

$$r^h(t+\alpha, t+2\alpha) = \xi + \eta r^h(t, t+\alpha).$$

A test of this naive projection method requires data for three enumeration years.

V. Productivity differences reflect regional wage-rate differences:

$$x_j^h(t) = \xi + \eta w_j^h(t)$$

A cross-sector for j again provides the data.

These illustrative hypotheses may be too simple. If so, multiple regression can provide a more effective means for test. For example, consider the hypothesis that market shares are determined by size of producer, size of consumer, and distance. This hypothesis must be expressed as a multiple-regression equation:

$$a_j^{hk} = \xi + \eta_1 X_j^h + \eta_2 U_j^h + \eta_3 d^{hk}$$

where d^{hk} is a measure of the distance between h and k.

There are many hypotheses that may be subjected to test. The reader undoubtedly can extend the above list.

Simultaneous Equation Approaches. The projection framework described by equation 16 can be converted to an analytical scheme by the making of constancy assumptions similar to those used for input-output analyses. Assume that the parameters values for $(t+\alpha)$ are given; one possibility is that they equal the values realized during t. One can then determine income levels by the insertion of external-use and residual-income levels.

Equation 16 then can be interpreted as an interregional multiplier-type system. Income multipliers are defined with respect to each external-use level. The multiplier $\phi_j^{hk}(t)$ is defined as the change of income in region h resulting from a one-unit increase in the use of good j in sector k. The multipliers are linear:

$$\phi_j^{hk}(t) = \sum_{i=1}^{6} \gamma^{hi} \beta_j^k a_j^{ik}$$

where γ^{hi} is the element in the hth row and i^{th} column of the inverse given in equation 16.

7. OMISSIONS AND EXTENSIONS

The account variables presented in this paper do not represent a complete listing of all the data that are desirable for the analysis of regional growth. They merely represent a collection of data which the author believes would be of great value for regional analysis. Many other types of data would be of considerable value. If priorities are necessary for the collection of new data, it is the contention of this paper that flow, i.e., trade, data should receive a high priority.

The illustrations presented here represent only a few of many possible applications for data covering interregional trade and associated variables. Hopefully, the reader can supply many more.

The illustrations have also been limited to methods not far removed from those currently used in regional economics. A consideration of the usefulness of accumulated international-trade theory for interregional analysis represents the first step in evaluating the usefulness of interregional-trade information.

COMMENT

GEORGE H. BORTS
Brown University

Professor Henderson has very ably summarized the analytic framework underlying the research of the Upper Midwest Study

Group. The following comments are partly expository and partly critical. Where they are critical the reader should bear in mind that Henderson's work and the work of his group is first-rate. They have advanced our knowledge of regional economics.

Professor Henderson's framework relates the output of a region to that of the nation through the estimation of export multipliers. His model is a derivative of an open input-output framework, where the domestic interindustry portion of the matrix has been collapsed. He makes use of the trade sub-matrices which summarize commodity flows between regions.

The trade matrices are converted into a projective device by the assumption of numerical values for the following parameters:

a_j^{hk}, the market share enjoyed by region h when selling the jth good to region k

x_j^h, the value of shipments per worker in the jth industry of region h

w_j^h, the value of wage payments per worker in the jth industry of region h

v_j^h, the value of non-wage income per worker in the jth industry of region h

b_j^k, the share of income produced in region k devoted to expenditure on the jth good.

The numerical values assumed may be those estimated from current or past data. As Professor Henderson tells us, "Some parameters are assumed to remain unchanged, some are modified by *ad hoc* methods, and some are estimated from behavior equations." He also tells us, "If trade coefficients do not prove stable, information covering their values over time is even more important, since it will provide the wherewithal to investigate the nature of their change."

This approach raises two fundamental questions. If indeed the parameters are constant over time, then the income produced in the Upper Midwest region is a linear function of income produced in the other regions of the United States. Observations on income levels in the two sets of regions would provide us with the characteristics of this linear relation. Note that we could not identify the individual a, x, w, v, and b through this method, but it would not matter. For we would have as good a predictive device as could be obtained by individual measurement of trade flows and parameters. The question is: Why not do it this way; why go through the enormous bother of estimating the entries of a trade matrix, as well as large numbers of productivity coefficients? Presumably the answer is that the parameters are not constant and that projection based on constant parameters would lead to serious error.

This brings up the second question. If the parameters are not constant, how do they change? It is clear that they have changed in the past. Indeed many would argue that the process of economic development requires them to change. Yet there is no obvious relation between the growth of a region and the share of the jth market which it enjoys in the neighboring region.

What Henderson has provided is a formal framework for projecting regional output. We are not yet provided with the theory of regional development which tells us how to change the parameters of the framework. Until this is done, the usefulness of the framework to other investigators remains an open question. As I have pointed out, unless the parameters do change, the framework has little rationale.

I should now like to turn away from the trade and productivity parameters of Professor Henderson's framework and discuss the weak link between labor supply and regional growth. One cannot explain the growth of a region without showing how its labor force is provided and how the growth of the labor force affects the growth of output. I have a strong complaint concerning the treatment of labor in the present paper. The level of migration appears to be a slack variable. It appears to be determined by the numerical difference between potential and actual employment, adjusted for population-support coefficients. In this model, potential employment is presumably determined by the potential size of the population before migration and by labor-force-participation rates. Actual employment is determined by external demands for exports interacting with the coefficients of the trade structure and with certain average labor-productivity coefficients. In this framework, population is determined as the number of people who can be supported by actual employment plus a number of unemployed. Any excess population over this is defined to migrate. Thus there is no way in which an excess of potential over actual employment can lead to more growth. There is no way in which autonomous in-migration can lead to growth, and no way in which the elasticity of the labor supply or shifts in the labor supply can influence growth. Surely a framework of this sort is less than ideal for explaining growth in rapidly growing regions, where the supply of labor is heavily influenced either by migration or by interindustry shifts from low-wage sectors to high. I would venture the guess that the model as presented could not be applied successfully to the growth of the Minneapolis–St. Paul metropolitan area, which in large part may be explained by the inflow of labor from farming regions. If this model is to be applied to other regions, there must be allowance for the stimulating effects of migration.

I should like to summarize my view of Professor Henderson's model. He has shown a great deal of ability and ingenuity in its construction. It is a thoroughly developed and internally consistent export model. External-use levels of the region's exports determine the domestic level and composition of economic activity. Nevertheless, I feel it is a projective device that may lead the investigator astray out of failure to allow for many crucial elements of economic growth. There is no theory or explanation of a rise in output per worker; there is no transfer of resources to better-paying occupations; there is no relation between the elasticity of labor supply and the region's growth. Finally, and most important, the model portrays growth without ever investigating capital accumulation.

COMMENT

SIDNEY SONENBLUM
National Planning Association

Limited by the instructions of the Conference chairman to a paper on the use of flow accounts in regional analysis, Henderson has presented a straightforward trading model emphasizing the interregional movements of goods and services. Such a model is primarily useful for the analysis of short-term regional impact. In spite of the claims made for it, however, the model has less relevance to longer-term considerations even though it provides some opportunity to make interregional comparisons of growth and structure.

The building blocks in the Henderson flow account describe for each producing or consuming sector in a region its gross output, consumption, employment, income produced, population, and net migration. These building blocks are then combined into significant relationships, the principal ones of which are: trading coefficients relating sector output in one region to its use in another region; productivity coefficients relating sector output to employment in a given region; income coefficients relating sector income produced to employment in a given region; demand coefficients relating goods and services consumption to income received in a region; and population-support coefficients relating population to employment in a region.

There can be no doubt that in terms of their usefulness to a variety of regional problems, the feasibility of data-gathering, and their potential for contributions to cumulative regional research, Henderson has made an excellent selection of relevant variables. One might quibble with some of the specifics in the Henderson menu. For example: I sense that he is underestimating the difficulties of data-gathering, if such studies were made for each metropolitan area; it is surprising that he details sales to exogenous regions but not to the specific industries in other regions; and there is no indication of the serious conceptual and statistical difficulties in obtaining data on constant-dollar income produced.

However, being in no serious disagreement over details in this paper, I would like to take issue with the high priority assigned to gathering trading information. There seems to be a feeling that the most important gap in our regional data is the lack of information on interregional trading relationships. I don't believe that this is the case. A more serious gap, it seems to me, is the lack of regional information on public and private capital stock, on the size and skill of available manpower, and on the factors which induce people to migrate or remain where they are. Without the addition of stock and migration data, trading information would add little to "the art of regional projection" and a trading model would be little improvement over that standard whipping boy, the nation-to-region approach.

It seems to me that what is happening to the subnational economies is that regions are becoming more alike in their economic activities at the same time that interregional transactions are increasing in importance. These developments can occur together only if there is an increase in "cross-hauling." As Henderson points out, "cross-hauling" has no place in classical theory; this, of course, does not mean that it can be ignored. If the observed trading data show substantial cross-hauling, its "explanation" in terms of inefficient distribution or sector aggregation is not particularly informative. I suspect that some more basic phenomena are at work which are related to the highly urbanized and service economy to which we are becoming accustomed: an economy where non-commodity activities become export-oriented; where large population centers encourage manufacturing activities to become residentiary-oriented; where changing technologies require plants to produce for both export and residentiary markets; and where increased government activities encourage capacity location decisions to be made on the basis of such things as the unemployment characteristics of the regional work force.

The relevance of these illustrations is that we should not expect significant improvements in long-term projections of regional activities from the model here presented. As Henderson says, "If adequate explanatory equations for key regional variables were available, a much refined projection methodology could be developed. However, such equations are currently in short supply." I am not convinced that interregional trade data are the primary source for increasing the supply of key equations.

REGIONAL INCOME ACCOUNT ESTIMATES

EDWIN F. TERRY
Federal Reserve Bank of Kansas City

This paper consists of some general observations about preparing and assessing estimates of regional income accounts. These observations stem from a study of the documentation by the Office of Business Economics, U.S. Department of Commerce, of their efforts in estimating state personal income. Their estimating methods are applied here to the preparation of any income account for any region. The word "region" will be used to mean any subnational area.

1. OFFICE OF BUSINESS ECONOMICS REGIONAL ESTIMATES

The first regional income accounts published by the Office of Business Economics (OBE) that generally conformed to national accounts were those dealing with personal income by states, 1929–54, appearing in the September 1955 issue of the *Survey of Current Business*.[1] Since then, estimates have been published in the August issues; preliminary figures were released in the April 1961 and 1962 issues. Estimates of state disposable income also have been released. Other regional estimates conforming to national income

---

[1] August 1954 was the last date on which estimates of a series called "state income payments" were released by the Office of Business Economics. As noted by it, this series did not conform with present national income accounts. See "State Payments in 1949," *Survey of Current Business*, 30 (Aug. 1950), 11–24.

accounts have not been published by the OBE, although it has given assistance to groups preparing, for example, income estimates by counties.[2]

The economic composition of the state personal-income estimates will be indicated briefly. Basically, "State personal income is the current income received by residents of the States from all sources, inclusive of transfers from government and business but exclusive of transfers among persons," according to the OBE.[3] Income from all sources includes imputed income such as property income withheld by life-insurance companies on the account of policy-holders and net rental value of owner-occupied dwellings. Transfers among persons are omitted principally because of a lack of suitable data with which to estimate the state net balance.[4]

The category "state resident" is defined as consisting primarily of people who physically reside in a given state. The definition is not based on any notion such as usual, permanent, or legal residence, except for tourists or others who are in a state for a very temporary stay.[5] It excludes the wages and salaries of U.S. citizens working for the U.S. Government in foreign countries from state personal income and includes those of foreign-citizen employees of foreign governments working in the United States. These amounts are accorded the reverse treatment in national personal income because of the particular definition of "resident" used in its compilation.[6]

The resident category also includes what are termed "quasi-individuals." These consist of private non-profit institutions, private pension, health, and welfare funds, and private trust funds.[7] Private non-profit institutions include religious, labor, welfare, and relief organizations. The incomes of these organizations and funds are allocated among the states and included as part of their personal

---

[2] *Personal Income by States since 1929*, 1956 supplement to *Survey of Current Business*, p. 56.
[3] *Ibid.*, p. 57.
[4] *Ibid.*, p. 59.
[5] *Ibid.*, pp. 57–58.
[6] *National Income*, 1954 supplement to *Survey of Current Business*, p. 32, and *U.S. Income and Output*, 1958 supplement to *Survey of Current Business*, p. 201.
[7] *Personal Income* supplement, p. 59.

property income. They are included in personal income partly because additional data would be required to establish a separate sector for them and partly because they either serve individuals directly or are established in their behalf.[8] Although corporate farms are not classed as quasi-individuals, their income is included in the net-farm-income component of proprietor income. This situation arises from data difficulties.[9]

The major categories of personal income for the United States, with 1955 data included as an example, are:

	(in millions)
Wages and salaries	$208,039
Other labor income	7,136
Proprietors' income	41,421
Property income	37,690
Transfer payments	17,471
Less personal contributions for social insurance	5,155
Personal income	$306,598

Note: There is an official rounding error of plus $4 million in the components.
Source: "Personal Income by Major Sources, 1954–57," *Survey of Current Business*, 38 (Aug. 1958), p. 14.

Each of the various categories of personal income is estimated on a state basis as the summation of separately estimated components. Because of data difficulties, various categories of personal income—principally wages and salaries, and proprietors' income—include contributions to social-insurance funds. As a result, these contributions are estimated separately and included as a negative category of personal income by OBE. The question of interest is: How does it estimate these components? Excluding net farm-proprietor income, its estimating methods were found to be classifiable into five types of estimators from information contained in the 1956 *Personal Income* supplement to *Survey of Current Business*.[10]

[8] *Ibid.*, pp. 58–60.
[9] *Ibid.*, p. 117.
[10] In some cases, recourse to additional materials cited in the supplement was necessary for the classification. The information there is still relevant, for the reader is referred to that publication for statistical derivation of current estimates in the Aug. 1962 *Survey of Current Business*, p. 11.

The five estimator classifications used by OBE were: (1) estimates utilizing direct comprehensive data, (2) estimates utilizing direct data but on a sample inference basis, (3) estimates made by extrapolating benchmarks with proxy data, (4) estimates made by allocating national estimates according to the state relative share of some additive proxy variable total, and (5) estimates made by extending the state relative share of a national total at some prior benchmark period into subsequent time periods. The "direct data" referred to in the first two classifications means data which are an actual measure of the type of income whose regional total is being estimated. An additional requirement for the direct-data estimators is that such data be of annual or more frequent occurrence, that it relate to the year in question, and that it be regionally oriented. The last three estimators will be illustrated, in numerical order, by examples.

Very few direct data are available on year-to-year movements of state non-farm-proprietor income.[11] For this reason, OBE makes use of other data in making the proprietor-income estimates. State retail-trade-proprietor income, for example, is estimated by extrapolation of state benchmarks by retail-trade-employee payrolls.[12] The extrapolation process assumes a linear homogeneous regression relationship between proprietor income and payrolls. The sum of the state estimates is then adjusted to conform to independent estimates of national retail-trade-proprietor income. The state benchmarks are estimated from direct data from the Census of Business and the Internal Revenue Service. Inasmuch as employee earnings are not an actual measure of proprietor income, this estimator is classed in the "benchmark proxy extrapolator" category.

The "additive proxy allocator" will be illustrated by the method used to make state estimates of military pay receipts. Records of military disbursements are not maintained on a state basis.[13] The estimated annual cash pay received by military personnel in the states is allocated geographically in accordance with the number of persons assigned to duty stations within each state. This allocation

---

[11] *Personal Income* supplement, p. 103.
[12] *Ibid.*, p. 110.
[13] *Ibid.*, p. 52.

is made separately for officers and enlisted men by branch of service.[14] Number of personnel is not definitionally the same as cash pay; therefore data concerning it are not direct data. Benchmarks are not utilized. Number of personnel by states is a total quantitative characteristic and hence the state figures are meaningfully additive. Therefore, this particular estimator is classed as an "additive proxy allocator."

It will be noted that the word "proxy" is common to the last two estimators that have been discussed. This word will be explained briefly. The use of an auxiliary variable in estimators is well established in statistics.[15] However, the use of an auxiliary-variable estimator demands that some direct measurements be made of the characteristic being estimated. When this is not the case, then the auxiliary variable ceases to be auxiliary to, and becomes a substitute for, that characteristic. At this point, such a use of data prompts a change in name from "auxiliary" to "proxy." The extrapolator and allocator estimators have this quality in common; therefore the word "proxy" appears in both.

The "benchmark extension" estimator calls for application of the state relative distribution in a benchmark period to national totals to make state estimates in later periods. For example, national totals of the state and local government interest component of property income are allocated according to the state relative distribution at the time of a prior benchmark.[16]

OBE refers to three classes of estimator in its *Personal Income* supplement. They are (a) direct comprehensive, (b) allocation, and (c) benchmark extrapolation.[17] The last two are sometimes referred to as indirect.[18] Its "allocation" class consists of the previously defined benchmark extension estimator as well as the additive proxy allocator. This is indicated by its discussion of the state estimates of state and local government interest paid to persons.[19] Its benchmark extrapolator title includes the previously defined direct

[14] *Ibid.*, p. 97.
[15] William G. Cochran, *Sampling Techniques* (New York: John C. Wiley & Sons, 1953), Chs. 6 and 7.
[16] *Personal Income* supplement, p. 125.
[17] *Ibid.*, pp. 50, 51, and 69–70 respectively.
[18] *Ibid.*, p. 107.
[19] *Ibid.*, p. 125.

sample estimator as well as the benchmark proxy extrapolator as indicated in its discussion of the state estimates of farm wages and salaries.[20] The benchmark extension and direct sample estimator classifications are of relevance because their data requirements (and generally the estimates they would produce) are different from those of estimators with which they have been paired by OBE.

So that a quantitative, as well as qualitative, appraisal of OBE estimation methods could be presented, the amounts of personal income determined by each of the five estimators were estimated for 1955. The reason the word "estimated" is used is that some splits of personal-income data were required for the estimator classification that were not found in any publications and had to be estimated by the writer. The year 1955 was selected in preference to 1961 mostly because more data were available for the earlier year. Other data found only in the *Personal Income* supplement and relating to earlier years were judged to be put to less strain for 1955 than for later year estimates. It is noted that 1929 was the only year common to all the tabular data in the "Sources and Methods of Estimation" section of the supplement. The relative amount of personal income estimated by each of the five methods, excluding the net farm income of farm proprietors, was:

Direct comprehensive	56
Benchmark proxy extrapolator	21
Additive proxy allocator	13
Direct sample	8
Benchmark extension	2
	100

The non-farm personal-income components to which these figures refer constituted 96 to 97 per cent of aggregate state personal income in 1955 and subsequent years.

Some detail on the quantification of the 1955 personal-income-estimator classifications is shown in Table 1. In this table the three estimators not utilizing direct data, earlier identified as 3, 4, and 5, are summed into one category called "indirect." So, the 1955 per-

[20] *Ibid.*, pp. 76–77.

TABLE 1. Gross Components, U.S. Total of State Personal Income, 1955
(Excluding Alaska and Hawaii)
(in millions of dollars)

	Estimation method		
	Direct data		
Source	Comprehensive	Sample	Indirect
Wages and salaries			
Mining			
Construction			
Manufacturing			
Transportation except [a]	148,082		8,469
Communication and public utilities	(UI)		(BOASI)
Trade except [b]			
Finance, insurance, and real estate except [c]			
Services except [d]			
Railroad transportation			5,627
Water transportation			763
[a] Local electric railroads	63		
Services allied to Transportation, minor portion			76
[a b d] Tips			876
Federal Credit Unions	17		
Federal Reserve Banks	77		
[c] New Jersey Federal Reserve System members			60
Commission insurance solicitors			431
Private households			2,933
Private hospitals	962		241
[d] Private education, major portion			1,251
Non-profit organizations, major portion	435		1,195
Farm		2,622	85
Federal civilian	9,670		141
Federal military			7,495
State and local government		15,992	
Other industries	159		317
Other labor income			
Employer contribution to private pensions, etc.			5,383
Compensation for injuries	1,058		
Pay of military reservists	188		281
Other			226
Proprietors' income			
Non-farm proprietor			29,654
Farm gross income	229	31,659	1,741
Less farm production expenses		7,567	14,295
Property income			37,690

TABLE 1. Gross Components, U.S. Total of State Personal Income, 1955 (Excluding Alaska and Hawaii) (Continued)

(in millions of dollars)

	Estimation method		
	Direct data		
Source	Compre-hensive	Sample	Indirect
Transfer payments			
BOASI		4,915	
Federal Government life insurance	315		273
Federal civilian pensions	340		113
Other Federal transfers [1]	93		207
State and local government pensions	646		34
Business transfers			1,457
Military retirement			409
Mustering-out and terminal leave			297
UI	1,369		
Railroad benefits	713		
Veteran pensions and compensation	2,711		
Veteran allowances	723		
State and local government:			
Cash sickness compensation	63		
Direct relief	2,495		
Veteran aid and bonuses } Other transfers [2]	298		
Less personal contributions for social insurance			
BOASI			2,825
UI and cash sickness compensation	77		
Railroad retirement insurance			308
Federal civilian pension			502
State and local government pension	665		35
Government life insurance			445
Self-employed contributions	298		
Total	171,746	62,755	126,135
Percentage	48	17	35

[1] As defined in *Personal Income* supplement to *Survey of Current Business*, p. 133.
[2] *Ibid.*, p. 135.

UI = State unemployment insurance data.
BOASI = Bureau of Old Age and Survivors Insurance data.

Sources: *Personal Income by States since 1929*, 1956 supplement to *Survey of Current Business*; *U.S. Income and Output*, 1958 supplement to *Survey of Current Business*, pp. 170–71; and "Personal Income by Major Sources, 1954–57," *Survey of Current Business*, 38 (Aug. 1958), p. 14; with individual estimates by the author.

sonal-income components are shown by direct-comprehensive-data, direct-sample-data, and indirect-data estimator classifications. The stub of the table identifies varying aggregates of personal-income components estimated by OBE. Included in the components is farm-proprietor income classified according to its estimation by the two direct and one indirect estimator classifications. Net farm-proprietor income is estimated as the residual of farm gross income minus farm-production expenses. The gross components are estimated jointly by OBE and the Agricultural Marketing Service of the U.S. Department of Agriculture and are shown individually.

The amounts of the personal-income sectors, classified by the three estimation methods, are entered in the three figure columns of Table 1. The gross components indicated, without regard to algebraic sign, were estimated to total $360,636 million in 1955. Of this amount it was estimated that 48 per cent was derived from direct comprehensive data, 17 per cent was determined by sample infer-

TABLE 2. U.S. Total of State Personal Income, 1955 (Excluding Alaska and Hawaii)

(in millions of dollars)

Categories	Estimation method		
	Direct data		Indirect
	Comprehensive	Sample	
Wages and salaries	159,465	18,614	29,960
Other labor income	1,246		5,890
Proprietors' income	48	8,318	33,055
Property income			37,690
Transfer payments	9,766	4,915	2,790
Personal contributions for social insurance	1,040		4,115
Total	171,565	31,847	113,500
Percentage	54	10	36

ence from direct data, and the remaining 35 per cent was estimated by use of the indirect estimators previously illustrated. In the wages and salaries section, data stemming from state unemployment insurance (UI) and Bureau of Old Age and Survivors Insurance (BOASI) are identified. The Bureau of Old Age and Survivors Insurance figure was classified in the "indirect" category primarily because the data used for the estimator of industry earnings not covered by unemployment insurance in 1955 related to 1951.[21]

An allocation of the 1955 net-farm-income figure, according to the estimator classification of the farm gross components of Table 1, was performed. The substitution of the net-farm-income residual for the gross figures would cause the classification sectors in Table 1 to correspond in aggregate to the personal-income categories published by OBE. These results are shown in Table 2. The increase in the "comprehensive" and decrease in the "sample" percentages are caused by the decreased size in the Table 2 total of the farm component, which relies to a large degree on sample data.

2. ACCURACY OF PERSONAL-INCOME ESTIMATES

But how accurate are these estimates? This is a question that must be answered. The accuracy investigation will be confined to that portion of state personal income consisting of wages and salaries covered by unemployment insurance. OBE secures most of the data for these estimates from payroll tabulations of firms covered by the various state unemployment-insurance laws, compiled on a Standard Industrial Classification basis.[22] In speaking of its state personal-income estimates OBE has said, "Principally, though not solely, because of these unemployment insurance tabulations, the quality of the state wage and salary totals has improved to the point where it can be rated as generally excellent." [23]

The unemployment-insurance data is oriented regionally so that it reflects the state where employees work, which is not necessarily the state where they reside.[24] In conformity with the requirements of personal-income and disposable-income accounts, the wage and salary components should be on a residence (where received) basis. In making state personal-income estimates, OBE has indicated that it makes residence adjustments on a continuing basis to the where-employed private wage and salary data for nine states and the

[21] *Personal Income* supplement, p. 73.
[22] Technical Committee on Industrial Classification, Office of Statistical Standards, *Standard Industrial Classification Manual* (Washington, 1957).
[23] *Personal Income* supplement, p. 71.
[24] *Ibid.*, p. 52.

District of Columbia. The states adjusted are Maryland, Virginia, Kentucky, Ohio, Indiana, Illinois, New York, New Jersey, and Connecticut.[25] For the other 39 contiguous continental states, it assumes that the unemployment-insurance and other place-of-employer disbursement data on private wages and salaries furnish a close approximation to the employees' state of residence. Their statement is, "While this assumption cannot be tested in a wholly satisfactory way, the degree of error which it causes in state personal income is believed to be very small." [26]

The most obvious way to determine the accuracy of the state-covered estimates of wages and salaries received would be to compare them to the true values. Since the true values are not known, a different tack must be tried. The procedure will be to examine the estimator for formal (assumption) errors. If none can be demonstrated, all errors must be attributed to reporting discrepancies.

OBE does not make any residence correction to its unemployment-insurance data for Kansas and Missouri. To find that covered private wages and salaries earned in Missouri are entirely attributed to Missouri residents is somewhat disconcerting to a person acquainted with the Kansas City area. The reason for concern is that, on net balance, a considerable portion of the Kansas residents of the Kansas City Standard Metropolitan Statistical Area (KCSMSA), consisting of four counties, two in each state,[27] are commonly regarded as employed in Missouri. The question is how to test objectively the opinion concerning the Kansas net out-commuting.

Such a test has been made. The first problem was to obtain data on commuting. A list indicating the residence of the 684 employees on the payroll of the Kansas City, Missouri, main office of the Federal Reserve Bank of Kansas City in September 1962 was compiled. The list indicated that 21 per cent of these Kansas City, Missouri, employees lived in Kansas. This percentage was taken as representative of the gross Missouri in-commuting of Kansas residents. To estimate a commuting percentage net of Missouri residents commuting to jobs in Kansas, the following device was employed. First,

[25] *Ibid.*, pp. 100–2.
[26] *Ibid.*, p. 52.
[27] Redefined to include an additional county in Missouri as of Jan. 1, 1962.

the 1960 KCSMSA average wage and salary employment figure was divided by the corresponding 1960 population as indicated in the 1960 Census of Population. (KCSMSA non-agricultural wage and salary employment is estimated by the Missouri Division of Employment Security in cooperation with the U.S. Department of Labor. The Kansas Division of Employment Security publishes figures on the Kansas component. These figures are prepared on a where-employed basis.) Second, the resulting employment-participation-rate quotient was multiplied by the state population components of the KCSMSA, to give estimates of the number of employed residents in the state components. Third, the number of persons employed in the Missouri portion minus the estimated number of employed Missouri residents was positive and represented the Missouri net in-commuter estimate. The in-commuters amounted to 14 per cent of persons employed in the Missouri portion of the KCSMSA, a figure lower than the previous gross estimate of 21 per cent. This discrepancy was as anticipated. If the net percentage estimate had not been lower than the gross, considerable doubt would have been raised about this estimating procedure.

Before proceeding further, it was necessary to determine if the rest of Kansas would have an appreciable net interstate-commuter balance. A determination was made by inspection of a map of Kansas and its surrounding states. While such a judgment is hard to defend, it is guessed that if a net commuter balance exists for the rest of Kansas, it may very well be a Kansas-resident out-commuter balance. The following calculations take the Kansas net interstate-commuter balance, except in the two KCSMSA counties, to be zero.

To adjust the 1960 Kansas state personal-income figure for the estimated Kansas-resident net out-commuter balance, the following calculations were performed. The Kansas non-agricultural wage and salary net out-commuter figure was divided by Missouri state 1960 non-agricultural wage and salary employment. The resulting figure of approximately 3 per cent was multiplied by the OBE 1960 estimate of the Missouri private wage and salary component of personal income and yielded a wage and salary figure earned by Kansas residents attributed to Missouri of approximately $165 million. This figure, added to the OBE 1960 estimate of the Kansas wage and salary component of personal income, caused the total and percapita personal-income figures to increase by approximately 3.7 per cent. (It is noted that the OBE residence adjustments for New York and Connecticut have been 2.5 and 3 per cent of their personal-income totals, respectively, in the past.[28]) The Kansas 1960 per-capita-income figure increased from $2,057 to $2,133 or from 93 to 96 per cent of the U.S. average. The effect on the rank of Kansas among states in personal income per capita cannot be determined, because the effect of a residence adjustment for the other unadjusted states was not estimated. This particular residence adjustment to the OBE estimate of Kansas personal income is quite rough and should not be taken as indicating a proposed revised figure. A more accurate method of adjusting wages and salaries for the interstate commuter in all states is possible and will be described in the following paragraph.

As stated earlier, OBE obtains state summary tabulations, by place of employment for Standard Industrial Classification groups, of total wages paid to employees covered by unemployment insurance. An adjustment for state of residence of the earnings so reported is not possible from this data. However, the state unemployment-insurance agencies, commonly referred to as the State Employment Services or Employment Security Divisions, must maintain records by names of individuals so as to be able to implement the unemployment-insurance-benefits program. With names of individuals available it would be possible, so far as the data being compiled are concerned, to make a rather accurate estimate of interstate wage and salary commuters. That is, for known or possible interstate commuting areas, the individuals employed in those areas covered by unemployment insurance could be allocated as to state of residence by collation with telephone books, Internal Revenue Service tax returns, or state-income-tax returns. Not only might the numbers of wage-and-salary-worker state commuters covered by unemployment insurance be determined but, instead of a pro-rata estimate, their actual wages might be determined by recourse to the unemployment-insurance individual wage records.

The whole process of adjustment of commuter figures by re-

[28] *Personal Income* supplement, p. 102.

course to unemployment-insurance data could, of course, be performed on a sample basis. Some initial checking might disclose that some areas of interstate commuting would be quite stable and need only infrequent checks. The suggested method would be more direct than those utilized by OBE in which residence adjustments are made.[29]

It might not be amiss at this point to indicate that using unemployment-insurance data for both where-earned and where-received economic indicators is equivalent to saying that where-earned is the same as where-received for the regions involved, despite any mental reservations on the part of the persons making the estimates. It so happens that for many states whose unemployment-insurance data are not adjusted by OBE, this is now being done. The unemployment-insurance-earnings data are used by OBE for a where-received indicator in 39 states while many state unemployment-insurance agencies use the employment data from the same tax reports to make where-earned employment benchmarks and interim revisions in their state employment series.[30] The state employment figures are a where-earned indicator because the unemployment-insurance data and current monthly sample employment figures are reported on an employer-establishment basis. The monthly employment sample information received by state Bureau of Labor Statistics cooperators is utilized by the Bureau of Labor Statistics of the U.S. Department of Labor in its national employment series. The national employment series compiled on a resident basis is prepared from data secured by the Bureau of the Census of the U.S. Department of Commerce in sample surveys of households and does not utilize unemployment-insurance data.

3. APPRAISAL OF INCOME-ACCOUNT ESTIMATES

A quantitative appraisal of the accuracy of all the components of personal income as estimated by OBE would be a large order for

[29] *Personal Income* supplement, pp. 100–2.
[30] Bureau of Labor Statistics, U.S. Department of Labor, *BLS-State Employment Statistics Manual*, Vol. 1, General Topics (Washington, March 1, 1948), p. 38, and *Current Employment Statistics Manual*, 2, Operating Guide (Washington, March 1958), 12-14.

any one user of its estimates to perform. A less formidable task would be to assess adequacy of the estimates. Adequacy in this context means that competent people are putting forth a good effort in preparing their estimates. Adequacy can then be regarded as a necessary, but not necessarily sufficient, condition in attaining accuracy. A final judgment as to adequacy must, of course, be relative to the demands of the user. An appraisal of adequacy is dependent upon the authors of regional income account estimates supplying documentation as to how their estimates are prepared. If it is not supplied, then the quality of their estimates must remain largely unknown.

Here are some criteria for appraising adequacy: The first item to look for would be statements indicating that the persons making the estimates knew the conceptual content of the income accounts they have estimated. In addition, a list of the specific sources of data used to estimate various income-account components would be needed. Statements as to the correspondence of the source-data content to the composition of the income-account component, and any adjustments made to better the correspondence, should apply to both direct and proxy data. (It is noted that OBE relies heavily on disaggregation to improve correspondence.) The quantitative importance of the estimators used should be indicated. If sample data are used, a general indication of the sampling method and size would be of value, as well as indication of the computed standard errors for random samples. An indication of the correspondence between estimates and benchmark data would be helpful in judging accuracy. A statement as to whether the regional estimates are forced to agree with independent national-income-account estimates should be looked for even if estimates are presented for regions which are not exhaustive of U.S. totals.

A collation was made in the *Personal Income* supplement of these suggested adequacy criteria and the OBE write-up of its state personal-income and disposable-income estimates. This indicated that all but two points were presented to the writer's satisfaction. A breakdown of the quantitative importance of estimators used, in the format of Table 1 for each estimator, would have been quite helpful. A more quantitative indication of the correspondence of estimates of benchmark proxy extrapolators to intermittent benchmarks would have been desirable instead of the qualitative assessment presented. The following statement, pertaining to the proxy extrapolation of state benchmarks of wage and salary payments to workers in private households, in terms of wages and salaries received by workers in the personal-services industry, is an example of the OBE comments: "Tests showed the personal services series to be a satisfactory index of changes in the relative state distribution of domestic service payrolls from one census based benchmark to the next."[31] There is some uncertainty as to what constitutes "satisfactory."

The comments of this section have been made from the viewpoint of a user of regional estimates. The last section turns to the estimation of regional income accounts.

4. ESTIMATING REGIONAL INCOME ACCOUNTS

Reasons for making estimates of income accounts can be roughly divided into two groups, one pertaining to time and one to area. Time considerations are important when earlier or more frequent estimates than those available are desired. Examples of the more frequent type of estimation are the monthly estimates of state personal income for the nation prepared by *Business Week* magazine and monthly estimates for states in the Ninth Federal Reserve District by the Federal Reserve Bank of Minneapolis. Area considerations are important when estimates for an area or areas either have been discontinued or have never been prepared. An example of the latter is the county estimates of "net effective buying income" prepared by *Sales Management* magazine. Net effective buying income as estimated by *Sales Management* is not quite the same as disposable income because, for example, it excludes the value of the change in net farm inventories which enters into disposable income.[32] Net effective buying income is, however, stated

---

[31] *Personal Income* supplement, p. 89.
[32] "Survey of Buying Power," *Sales Management*, 88 (May 10, 1961), 54.

to be equivalent to disposable personal income by *Sales Management*.[33]

In making estimates of income accounts for any one area, or region, a survey of regional economic transactors could be employed. This method was pioneered by Charles L. Leven in his Ph.D. thesis and is reported in an article, "A Theory of Regional Social Accounting," in a precursor of the *Journal of Regional Science*.[34] This method would become rather expensive for any one organization to follow for all regions in the United States, particularly on a recurring basis. If field surveys are not made, then reports of government and private organizations must generally be relied upon for direct regional data and proxy measures with which to make income-account estimates. The question then arises as to which of the five estimators one would use to estimate a particular component of a regional income account, the five referred to being those used by OBE in estimating the non-farm components of state personal income.

From the standpoint of expected accuracy, the comprehensive and sample direct-data estimators would be preferred to the three indirect estimators. The choice between a comprehensive basis and a sample basis for the direct data would ordinarily be in favor of the former, to avoid sampling variability. The category of direct data, however, has been defined so that its regional orientation could be toward either income produced or income received. In the case of personal and disposable income, accounts must be compiled on the basis of the area of residence of the income recipient. Sample data on an income-received basis might be preferred to comprehensive data on an income-produced basis. The choice would depend upon the amount of discrepancy for a particular area and the ease of adjusting the comprehensive data to a received basis.

It should be noted that the income accounts nominally larger than personal income can be compiled on either a regional income-produced or a regional income-received basis.[35] A choice as to

---
[33] *Ibid.*, p. 56.
[34] *Papers and Proceedings of the Regional Science Association*, 4 (1958), 221-37.
[35] The difference may be called the "net in-area factor owner flow." A rigorous demonstration of the difference between factor earnings produced

which basis is to be used must be made and a strict conceptual adherence to it maintained.

If current direct data were not available, then an indirect estimator would have to be employed in estimating an income-account component. Of the three that have been discussed, the two utilizing area benchmarks would be more reassuring to use, as occasional indications of accuracy would be present. An empirical decision criterion for the choice between the benchmark-extension and proxy-extrapolator estimators would be past accuracy comparisons. This criterion would require benchmarks for two or more time periods so that estimates from one to the following could be checked for accuracy. The same criterion could be used in selecting the proxy variable with which to extrapolate a benchmark. If only one benchmark is available, the choice of proxy variable extrapolation or benchmark extension must be a matter of judgment. Because the regional relative share of the national total of an income component may vary over time, the proxy extrapolator appears to be structurally superior to benchmark extension because it is capable of admitting a changed relative share. If the estimates of a benchmark proxy extrapolator are to conform to national totals, then estimates must be prepared for all regions and forced to conform. If an estimate is desired for only a few regions and the remaining regions are combined, aggregation effects probably will be present.

If direct data and benchmarks were not available, the additive proxy allocator would have to be used. The choice of what variable to use as a proxy allocator must be a matter of judgment. This is because there are no independent checks on the resulting regional estimates. Such estimates would, by definition, have met the only

---

and those received in a given area is achieved by the following device. Consider: Income produced by factors employed in (out of) an area whose owners reside in (out of) the area. Four combinations of in and out are possible. The three income combinations relevant to a given area are: (1) in in, (2) in out, and (3) out in. The (2) combination, for example, is read: Income produced by factors employed *in* an area whose owners reside *out* of the area. The most meaningful area totals are the following: Income produced $= (1) + (2)$, income received $= (1) + (3)$, and net in-area factor owner flow $= (3) - (2)$. The difference between income received and income produced calculated from these totals is $(1) + (3) - [(1) + (2)] = (3) - (2) \times$ net in-area factor owner flow. Therefore, area income received $=$ area income produced $+$ net in-area factor owner flow, where net in-area factor owner flow can be positive or negative.

possible statistical check, namely that the sum of estimates for regions which are exhaustive of the United States conform to the U.S. total.

It is the general absence of independent data with which to check the accuracy of regional-income-account estimates that obliges the authors to document estimates that are published for use by others. Without documentation along the lines of the adequacy criteria suggested earlier, an assessment of regional estimates by such users must remain extremely primitive.

COMMENT

RUTH P. MACK
Institute of Public Administration

National income, regional income, state income, and the income of minor subdivisions share the characteristic that they can never be known. They can only be estimated. By and large, the percentage error of the estimates is likely to be smaller for larger than for smaller geographic entities. Terry discusses two sorts of hurdles that regional estimation must surmount. Both are aggravated, the second one particularly, by progressive geographic subdivision. But Terry hopes, very sensibly, by examining problems at the state level to learn something of how best to deal with them for smaller subdivisions.

The first problem is the absence of better rather than poorer methods of estimation. He classifies the methods that are used by the Office of Business Economics into five groups—direct comprehensive, direct but sample, benchmark proxy extrapolators, additive proxy allocators, benchmark extensions. He seems to feel that the prima facie evidence for adequacy deteriorates as one moves down this list.

Yet I doubt that the labels necessarily imply a grading system.

Consider, for example, the controversy that has raged in high places concerning whether sample surveys are more or less reliable than "comprehensive" censuses. Benchmark proxy extrapolators can provide excellent estimates when benchmark and proxy are suitable and sound. The awful truth about evaluating estimates is that it is as much work to evaluate them as to make them in the first place, perhaps more. A companion truth for short-cut methods that may be required for regional estimates is that there are no rules for bridging gaps in data except to use the best information and techniques available in each particular case.

The second problem that Terry examines is that of allocating wage and salary income on a where-received rather than where-earned basis. Of course, some of the difficulties have in practice been reduced by the use of the social-security wage and salary data as a "benchmark allocator" for census statistics. Terry weighs the magnitude of the problem by assembling some information on travel patterns. The 1960 Census, which questioned people concerning where they worked, provides a potential source for comprehensive analysis of this problem.

Needless to say, there is endless room for useful work in improving and preparing regional income accounts. However, the very endless character of the problem implies that the end is not automatic. It must be chosen. And a good choice in economic research is no different from other economic choices—it involves maximizing marginal yields. I submit that one important criterion of the marginal yield of research time and effort concerns the *question* to which the research is addressed. Terry is interested in the broad question of essaying interregional economic welfare. And certainly this is a matter of high importance. But for the question to be made more productive it must be narrowed somewhat, and one way this is often done is by choice of a level of concern: does interest in economic welfare focus on *description* of differences in welfare, in *analysis* of their causes, or in judging and formulating public *policy*?

Work on national income accounts for regions has the great advantage of not having to break entirely new ground. The long history of work with national income estimates for this country and for an increasing number of other countries has exposed all sorts of uses to which the information may be put. In this respect the history of national income estimates has paralleled that of other vast statistical compilations. There appears to be a sort of life cycle to these mammoth edifices of data. They may be whistled into being by some analytic use of almost hypothetical figures, but they begin primarily in the context of description. The acceptance as a partner in full standing of their value as analytic instruments, tools for the understanding of relationships and process, comes later. In the case of the income-expenditure survey, it came in the National Resources Committee Survey of 1935-36. The flow-of-funds account has not yet penetrated very far into stage two—analysis; it seems to have jumped to stage three in the limited context of banking policy. For national income and product measures the process was gradual. The twenties witnessed the period of gestation in which description was the most that could be achieved. But in the thirties, spurred on by Lord Keynes' powerful theorizing, income and product accounts became instruments of analysis and policy; they have continued increasingly in this role since. International comparisons, and the development of statistical measures of national income for most countries of the world, have proceeded at all three levels at an accelerating pace since the war. The regional income account, learning from the history of international comparisons, can start grown up and deal without delay with the matters of analysis and policy on which it can throw light.

Yet if this occurs, the priorities in data collection will be very different with respect to the definition of region and the character of data from what they would be if comprehensive and accurate description were the prime concern. For one thing, policy involves a capability for action, and this in many contexts rests with governments. Accordingly, "regions" must be defined as political jurisdictions, small as well as large, even though flexibility to cope with political overlays may be achieved.

Interest in process and policy likewise emphasizes the content of measurement. Government services, for example, are a form of goods dealt out without expense to the user; his matching expense is taxes paid. But unlike most purchases of goods, the matching does not take place at the level of the consumer unit nor even at the level of small or even larger regions. It differs for several major classes of governmental services and tax payments. In consequence it is important to know the size of the net balance and its composition for regions. A second example of interregional differences important in analyzing process and policy concerns the size distribution of incomes. An experiment indicates that relative income inequality is greater in low-income than in high-income states. To be specific, in the five states having the largest median family income according to the 1950 Census of Population, 60 per cent of the families had incomes within ±50 per cent of the median income. In the five states having the lowest median income only 38 per cent of the families were in the relatively-equal-income group. This tentatively suggests that regional differences in relative income distribution may be large and tend to exacerbate interregional contrasts in average incomes.

These examples do no more than illustrate the backlog of questions focusing on process and policy to which regional income accounts might be addressed. They suggest that the opportunity costs of refining double-entry income and product accounts are high. If these problem-oriented measurements are taken as serious competitors for the scarce resources of talent, diligence and enthusiasm, and even money, there might be an argument for some withdrawal from refinement of interlocked double-entry coverage. Instead the rich detail of employment, production, sales, personal-income, and other data available by local areas could be refined and exploited in response to important questions urgently in need of expert answers.

COMMENT

CHARLES E. FERGUSON
Duke University

The Millingtons are delighted with their new home which Deedee describes as "typical Connecticut—a gray shingle house" on a large piece of property. She describes Fairfield as a true country com-

munity more like Wayne than any other Chicago suburb. "We love it though it will take John three days to get to his office," she notes of the long commuter trip to Rockefeller Center. . . .
—*Chicago Daily News*

And then comes the long weekend, and the drinking.
—*The New Yorker*

So long as there are boundaries there will be commuters. The situs problem is an old one that has never had a very satisfactory solution from the standpoint of empirical implementation. The commuter-adjustment proposal contained in the paper under review seems to fail on this very ground. That is, the suggested treatment of the situs problem entails such a vast amount of clerical and statistical work that it seems prohibitively expensive.

There are two aspects of the paper to which I shall address remarks. The first, and more important, concerns the proposed method for revising state income data to represent "where received" rather than "where earned" personal income. Briefly, the method is as follows: obtain the names of all employees covered by unemployment insurance; determine their state of residence by "collation with telephone books, Internal Revenue Service tax returns, or state-income-tax returns"; adjust state income data for commuters by using the individual wage records of those covered by unemployment insurance.

My objections to this method are twofold. First, a large segment of the commuting population is excluded. Second, and perhaps more important, the magnitude of the task would be enormous. If such an expensive program is to be undertaken, one could presumably achieve greater accuracy by complete tabulation of income data from individual W-2 forms and from individual declarations of estimated income.

The second criticism concerns the specific Kansas-Missouri commuter adjustment. Let E, P, and N represent employment, population, and state population components of the Kansas City Standard Metropolitan Statistical Area (KCSMSA). Subscripts t, m, and k refer to total, Missouri, and Kansas data, respectively. The adjustment process, given the available data, is as follows:

(1) $\quad \dfrac{E_t}{P_t} =$ employment participation coefficient; so

(2) $\frac{E_t}{P_t}N_m$ = estimated number of Missouri residents employed in KCSMSA.

E_t and E_k are tabulated, so:

(3) $$E_t - E_k = E_m.$$

Thus

(4) $$E_m - \frac{E_t}{P_t}N_m = C_k,$$

where $C_k > 0$ is the estimated number of net commuters from Kansas into Missouri. Let T_m and Y_m represent total Missouri employment and the OBE estimate of the Missouri wage and salary component of personal income. Hence

(5) $$\frac{C_k}{T_m}Y_m = \text{Kansas income adjustment.}$$

The process just described does yield an adjustment for Kansas personal income, under the assumption that the rest of Kansas (outside the KCSMSA) has a zero commuter income balance. But there are other assumptions embodied in the calculation process as well. In the first place, one must assume that the employment participation coefficient is the same for the K and M areas. This may or may not be true; but generally it would not hold if one of the state areas were primarily residential, the other primarily commercial and industrial.

However, if the assumption is valid, (2) gives an estimate of the number of Missouri residents employed in the KCSMSA. Therefore, given an independent tabulation of E_k, (4) gives the estimated number of net Kansas residents commuting into Missouri (C_k). Finally, to obtain the correction factor embodied in (5), one must assume that the income per employee in the whole state of Missouri is equal to the income per employee in the KCSMSA.

If all these assumptions correspond to empirical reality, the estimated correction is an accurate representation of the wage-and-salary correction that should be made. However, since the assumptions are empirically so questionable, I doubt that this particular estimate is itself empirically useful. In addition, the correction is made only for wage-and-salary employees.

The situs problem is a *problem*. It can be solved exactly if the governmental units involved decide it is worth the cost of solution. If state governments do not think the revisions worth their (opportunity) cost, I am personally willing to accept the (partially commuter-adjusted) OBE estimates of personal income by state. These estimates probably do not involve a greater distortion than that contained in the specific K–M adjustments. Furthermore, to the extent that commuting is relatively stable over time, the OBE time series yield accurate growth rates, because each item is systematically biased.

Finally, one should not overlook the fact that aggregate supply is just as important as aggregate demand. In the last analysis, a state that feels deficient in the former must do something more positive than data adjustment to solve its problems.

PUBLIC FINANCE AS AN INTEGRAL PART OF REGIONAL ACCOUNTS

JESSE BURKHEAD [1]
Syracuse University

Those who have worked in recent years at the development of regional concepts and at the measurement of regional economic activity are by this time aware that their efforts have no clearcut policy orientation. Regional accounting is not directed toward a set of regional policies nor toward an organizational structure, public or private, with responsibility for regional well-being. The measurement of levels of private economic activity within a region does not in any sense imply, for example, that there is or should be a regional trade policy or a regional development policy, a point which was well made by Werner Hochwald in his 1957 paper.[2] And, as Clark Bloom pointed out in his review of Walter Isard's *Methods of Regional Analysis*, there is no compelling problem that dominates the field of regional analysis to give it focus in the same way that economic stabilization has dominated macroeconomics and the monopoly problem has dominated microeconomics.[3]

The absence of policy orientation is particularly disturbing as one attempts to prescribe a system of accounts for the measure-

---

[1] This paper has benefited greatly from comments on an earlier draft by Joseph Berliner, Dick Netzer, Harvey Perloff, and Werner Hirsch.

[2] "Conceptual Issues of Regional Income Estimation," in National Bureau of Economic Research, *Regional Income*, Vol. 21 of *Studies in Income and Wealth* (Princeton: Princeton University Press, 1957), pp. 9–26.

[3] *American Economic Review*, June 1961, p. 432.

ment of government activity within a region. All accounting systems, public or private, are structured by the purposes that they are intended to serve. But what are the purposes served by the public finances of a region? There is, of course, no regional government with authority to define goals and objectives or to impose a regional rationality on public-sector behavior. Instead, in every region there is a multiplicity of governmental units, which often work at cross-purposes and with goals and programs that are in frequent conflict one with another.

Numbers of examples could be adduced to illustrate this point, but a few will suffice. Currently a great many central-city-government agencies are working toward a very specific goal—the restoration of the economic health of the central business district. This goal may be completely rational from the standpoint of downtown merchants but it may be somewhat less than rational from the standpoint of a metropolitan region as a whole. At the same time other government agencies in metropolitan areas, with support from the state and federal levels, are pursuing an objective that may likewise have some claim to rationality—the maximization of the private use of automobiles. Unfortunately, the maximization of automobile usage compounds the difficulties encountered in restoring the central business district and, in addition, throws off large chunks of social costs in other directions as well.

Seemingly rational goals and objectives are pursued by the governments of upper-income suburbs in efforts to provide substantial public amenities by way of recreation, transportation, public health, and public education. Many suburbs implement these efforts by satisfying a highly developed "taste for discrimination," to use Gary Becker's unhappy phrase.[4] Exclusionist practices abound. At the same time, the central city has rational goals and objectives—to eliminate slums, to combat delinquency and crime, to provide respectable housing for its citizens. The pursuit of these goals is made vastly more difficult by the practices of the exclusionist suburbs. That which is a variable for the suburb is a parameter for the central city. It may be possible to demonstrate, by the criteria

[4] *The Economics of Discrimination* (Chicago: University of Chicago Press, 1957).

of welfare economics, that in these circumstances both the central city and the suburb are worse off, but this kind of finding will not convince the exclusionists.

These conflicting rationalities make for particular difficulties in efforts to measure the elements that make up a "region's health and well-being." Werner Hirsch has suggested that there are five dimensions that can be identified here: per-capita real income, basic employment stability, net social benefits, economic growth, and amenities of life.[5] Hirsch, however, would be the first to admit that these dimensions are frequently in conflict, as, for example, when a community must sacrifice employment stability to achieve growth. Also, at any one time and place there are a great many other dimensions of regional health and well-being, such as the consolidation of political and economic power positions, that are determinative of public and private decisions.

There is considerable danger that a good deal of private economic development in any specific region and a substantial part of government activity associated therewith has as its goal and purpose the avoidance of payment for social costs. The continued presence of tax havens, residential and industrial; the suburban "white noose" around the central city; the subservience of government officials to the interests of motorized transport—these conditions would suggest that for the metropolitan region, at least, the definitions of regional purpose, regional goals, regional well-being, and regional rationality will continue to be most elusive.[6]

The absence of clearly defined regional goals for public policy makes it difficult to devise a set of public-finance accounts for a region. We are in considerable danger of imposing our own idealized patterns of measurement and our own assumptions about regularity

---

[5] Werner Z. Hirsch, "Design and Use of Regional Accounts," *American Economic Review*, May 1962, p. 366.

[6] The foregoing is a partial restatement of a view that has been advanced most strongly by Lewis Mumford. In *The City in History* (New York: Harcourt, Brace & World, 1961), Mumford describes the forces that are in control as "insensate." By this he apparently means not irrational but unfeeling. He finds that the development of our cities is at best haphazard, at worst chaotic and anarchic. To Mumford, research on metropolitan problems would simply reveal relative states of dysfunction. Mumford would probably feel that a system of regional accounts reflects an effort to find regularity where none in fact exists.

when in fact regional economic activity may be highly irregular. This danger is particularly acute as we move from descriptive schema to projections. It may be that the elements which are determinative of regional growth are not those which are reflected in regional accounts. Extraregional forces, including national policy; semiautonomous changes in technology, particularly as these affect transportation; the political power structure of a region—these influences and decision patterns may contain the elements for understanding regional growth and development and the public finances therein. Accounting structures are not equipped to handle such variables, particularly in an open economy.

One other reservation is in order before we turn to the subject at hand. As things now stand, there is a widening gap between the conceptual development of regional accounting techniques and the provision of the data necessary for implementation. Some, like Harvey Perloff, are optimistic that this gap will be closed in the next decade.[7] In the meantime, however, social scientists who are interested in regional accounting continue to push the conceptual frontier farther and farther beyond the data that are available. Simultaneously, those who are responsible for public and private decisions within the metropolitan area are handicapped by the absence of some very ordinary kinds of data. Annual estimates of county income received and produced, annual population estimates by municipality, data on assessed and equalized property values by class of property—all this is information that could be fed immediately into local decision processes. Its availability should bring substantial improvement in the quality of local decisions, particularly for the public sector, although it may be suspected that intelligent communities secure better data and that data per se will not make community leaders more intelligent. Nevertheless, in our zeal for conceptual development we should not overlook the possibilities for immediate improvement in the organization and collection of rudimentary data.[8]

[7] Harvey S. Perloff, *A National Program of Research in Housing and Urban Development* (Washington: Resources for the Future, Inc., 1961).

[8] One of the most promising developments is that now under way at RAND under the direction of Edward F. R. Hearle; see "A Data Processing System for State and Local Governments" (Santa Monica: The RAND Corporation, mimeo, 1962). The Unified Information System that is proposed here would

But, now that these reservations about regional rationality and the relationship of conceptual structures to available data have been expressed, such concerns will be put aside in favor of the subject at hand. We can be generally confident that the needs for comprehensive and co-ordinated reporting of governmental activities for metropolitan regions will increase and not diminish in the immediate future. The increased complexity of governmental structures and the increased dispersion of political authority will require additional policy co-ordination at the same time that the ability to co-ordinate diminishes.[9]

The remainder of the paper is divided into four sections. The first will examine briefly the manner in which the public sector has been treated in previously developed comprehensive regional accounting schemes. The second will examine some general conceptual problems related to the public finances. The third section will explore the purposes that may be served by the public-finance component of a regional accounting system. The paper will close with some observations on regional accounts and regional decisions.

1. THE PUBLIC SECTOR IN REGIONAL SOCIAL ACCOUNTS

The pioneering work on comprehensive regional accounting for interindustry transactions by W. W. Leontief, Walter Isard, and Leon Moses did not place special emphasis on the public sector. Government, in this framework, is treated as a final demand sector, and the major task is to assure that the revenue and expenditure of state and local governments are properly added to other sectors. This approach limits the data requirements for the model and is, of course, perfectly appropriate where emphasis is placed on the measurement of activity levels among sectors and between one region and the rest of the world.

---

greatly enhance the availability and analysis of state and local data, but it would not apparently comprehend, under present plans, data on federal-government activities in regions.

[9] For a recent and forceful statement of this point of view see Anthony Downs, "Metropolitan Growth and Future Political Problems," *Land Economics*, November 1961, pp. 311–20.

The same general approach has been used in more recent studies for metropolitan areas, for both input-output and income and product accounts. No effort has been made to introduce additional refinements into the government sector, nor indeed are they required for the purposes intended to be served by the accounts.

For example, in the Stockholm accounts, Artle employs five sectors: (1) production, (2) industries in the rest of Sweden, (3) foreign countries, (4) government authorities, (5) households.[10] The government-authorities sector has three components: (1) the city of Stockholm, (2) all other municipal authorities in the country, (3) the national government. Transfer payments are identified, and some areas of local government, such as education, are isolated as separate sectors. Artle was unable to separate the 28 small local governments in the Stockholm area, apart from the city of Stockholm, and therefore consigned them to the "all other" category.

The Stockholm accounts report somewhat more detail on revenue than other studies, set forth in a three-way classification: direct and indirect taxes, and income from property and entrepreneurship. The separation of the national government from other governments permitted Artle to report on what might be termed "the local balance of payments for national government activity." He found, interestingly enough, that Stockholm residents paid more to the national government than they got back.

The Hochwald-Striner-Sonenblum accounts for the local impact of foreign trade on Kalamazoo, Mobile, and Gloversville utilized a different and in some ways more restricted approach to the government sector.[11] Government as a final demand sector was defined as local government. For example, any state and federal activity in Kalamazoo County was classified as non-local. Local-government capital formation was included in gross private domestic capital formation. Local-government transfers, interest, subsidies, and surplus were not separately identified and were assumed to be zero.

[10] Roland Artle, *Studies in the Structure of the Stockholm Economy* (Stockholm: Business Research Institute, Stockholm School of Economics, 1959).
[11] See Werner Hochwald, Herbert E. Striner, and Sidney Sonenblum, *Local Impact of Foreign Trade: Technical Supplements* (Washington: National Planning Association, 1960).

The detail for the local-government receipts and expenditure account is as follows:[12]

Purchases of goods and services	—
Local goods and services	—
Manufacturing establishments	—
Other private establishments	—
Employee compensation and transfers	—
Non-local goods and services	—
Manufacturing	—
Other private establishments	—
Transfers, interest, subsidies, surplus	0
Total government expenditures	—
Personal tax and non-tax	—
Corporate and indirect business taxes	—
Transfers from non-local governments	—
Total government receipts	—

The supplementary study of the Kalamazoo County economy by Harold T. Smith sets forth the detail on local-government purchases from industry by type of industry, and on local-government revenue from industry by type of industry.[13] These are the data needed for an impact study; local-government activity levels are revealed but there is little information that will facilitate the analysis of government program levels.

The Hirsch accounts for St. Louis do not provide as much detail for local government as does either set of Kalamazoo County accounts, but they do distinguish, within final demand, among federal, state, and local governments. In one classification the St. Louis study puts a part of local government into the processing sector.[14]

The deWolff and Venekamp accounts for Amsterdam provide about the same degree of accounting refinement as the Stockholm

---

[12] *Ibid.*, Technical Supplement E, "Relationship of Local Accounts to Other Regional Accounting Systems," p. 23.

[13] Harold T. Smith, *The Kalamazoo County Economy* (Kalamazoo: Upjohn Institute for Employment Research, 1960), pp. 196–200.

[14] Werner Z. Hirsch, "The Economy of the St. Louis Area," in *Exploring the Metropolitan Community*, John C. Bollens, ed. (Berkeley: University of California Press, 1961), pp. 369–87, 460–82.

accounts.[15] The consolidated account of the Amsterdam government is as follows:

Payments:
Goods and services bought from enterprises
   in Netherlands and rest of world   —
To consumers at Amsterdam
   Wages and salaries (including social-
     insurance contributions)   —
   Incomes transferred   —
To consumers in rest of Netherlands   —
   Wages and salaries (including social-
     insurance contributions)   —
     Total   —

Receipts:
Goods and services rendered to:
   Enterprises at Amsterdam   —
   Consumers at Amsterdam   —
   Indirect taxes minus subsidies   —
   Direct taxes   —
   Interest and profits   —
     Total   —

Judged by the single criterion of the amount of public finance detail made available, the Stone-Deane regional accounts for Great Britain for 1948 are by all odds the most satisfactory.[16] Although these are cast in terms of input-output, the classification can most easily be described in income and product accounts.[17] In the regional product-expenditure account indirect taxes collected in the region are shown on the product side, and sales of goods and services to the central government on the expenditure side. The regional income and outlay account shows direct taxes on the outlay side and central-government transfers on the income side. The regional capital account distinguishes central-government

[15] P. deWolff and P. E. Venekamp, "On a System of Regional Social Accounts for the City of Amsterdam," *Bulletin de l'Institut International de Statistique*, 35 (Rio de Janeiro, 1957), 203-17.

[16] Richard Stone, "Social Accounts at the Regional Level: A Survey," in *Regional Economic Planning*, Walter Isard and John H. Cumberland, eds. (Paris: OEEC, 1961), pp. 263-95.

[17] Stylianos Geronymakis, "Discussion Paper," *ibid.*, pp. 297-303.

from private gross investment. There are a central-government current account and a central-government capital account, which detail the transactions between the region and the central government, and the appropriate consolidated accounts.

What the Stone-Deane accounts do, better than any other set that has yet been devised, is to spell out the pattern of transactions between the region and the central government. The accounts fail, however, to provide a complementary accounting scheme for local government within the region.

Those who have worked within an income and product framework for regional accounting have not been very much more generous in the treatment of the government sector. In his excellent paper at the first Conference on Regional Accounts, Leven was forthright in his examination of the difficulties encountered in measuring national and state government activity within the region; he then proceeded to amalgamate most of local government into the private sector.[18]

The public sector fares somewhat better in the Berman-Chinitz-Hoover projections for the New York metropolitan region.[19] Here government expenditure and employment are isolated and capital expenditures and government enterprise are not consolidated with the private sector. Federal employment is separated from state-local, and there are subsidiary classifications that distinguish capital outlay, payroll expenditures, and other. Government demand for the output of each of the 43 industries employed in the interindustry table is, of course, a part of the projections.

The fact that the regional accounting systems that have thus far been devised present only the most limited data for the government accounts is not, of course, a criticism of these systems. Regional accounts have simply not been designed with a view to the identification and analysis of government activity, or with a view to providing information significant for public policy decisions.

---

[18] Charles L. Leven, "Regional Income and Product Accounts: Construction and Applications," in *Design of Regional Accounts*, Werner Hochwald, ed. (Baltimore: The Johns Hopkins Press, 1961), esp. pp. 156-59.

[19] Barbara R. Berman, Benjamin Chinitz, and Edgar M. Hoover, *Projection of a Metropolis* (Cambridge: Harvard University Press, 1961), esp. pp. 21-22.

Nevertheless, the fact that these accounting systems are inadequate for a great many government decisions does suggest that some additional classifications must be added. Certainly the minimum requirements are the separate identification of federal, state, and local government activities and a distinction within each of these for capital outlay, other goods and services, and transfer payments. It would also be highly useful to distinguish among general government, trust funds, and public enterprise. But these are not the kinds of distinctions that fit well into an interindustry matrix. In this context government enterprise properly belongs to the processing sector, not to final demand, and the treatment of transfer payments as final demand is somewhat awkward. Moreover, the provision of this kind of detail for the public sector requires a type of disaggregation that serves no useful purpose for input-output.

Although the present writer is certainly not an expert in interindustry analysis, one conclusion would seem to him to be evident. This is that adequate information on the public finances of the region cannot easily be contained in an input-output matrix. The best hope would appear to lie in the development of a family of subsidiary statements linked with and fully integrated with comprehensive regional accounts but capable of standing on their own feet and useful for purposes quite different from those to which the integrated accounts may be put.[20]

2. THE CONCEPT OF GOVERNMENT IN A REGION

As the foregoing summary review indicates, we have now accumulated considerable experience in the treatment of local government in a system of regional accounts. The principal deficiencies, from a public finance–public policy standpoint, lie in the sparsity

[20] This point is reminiscent of the several-decades-old argument about a single set of accounts for the federal government. This argument appears to have been resolved in favor of multiple systems. The Council of Economic Advisers and the Bureau of the Budget now publish and discuss, in a policy-oriented framework, the conventional budget, the cash consolidated budget, and the income and product budget. Each of these can be reconciled with the income and product accounts.

of information typically presented. These deficiencies can be remedied by supplementary classifications.

A much more difficult problem is posed, both conceptually and in terms of data availability, by the presence of non-local government within the region. From a public-finance standpoint, however, the ideal treatment is clear. Non-local-government activity should be assigned to local areas, preferably to municipalities. This classification will permit a consolidated public-finance account for each municipal area, to show the expenditure of federal, state, and local governments therein and possibly the revenue derived therefrom. These municipal-area accounts can then, again ideally, be further consolidated into a government account for the entire region. This is the only technique by which it will be possible to secure a comprehensive view of the public finances of a region.

Regional accounting systems that are intended to measure economic-activity levels treat federal and state government activity within the region as a part of the rest-of-the-world sector. A regional governments account requires a quite different approach, with emphasis on the area in which federal and state expenditures are made rather than on the national or state-wide range of benefits.

Federal-government programs, for example, are sustained and promoted by a mixture of national, regional, and narrowly local considerations. National-defense expenditures, to use the standard polar case, do indeed provide a service for the nation as a whole, but there are regional dimensions as well. Specific areas are protected and there are economic-process effects from federal expenditures for national defense, just as for other federal expenditures. These process effects have very clear regional consequences, although for programs such as those in defense and international affairs it may not be possible to measure a level of regional benefits as distinguished from a level of regional expenditure.

Some federal expenditures are indissolubly linked with local economic-activity levels, as in the case of the Post Office Department. In other cases the existence of a national policy in such areas as those of agriculture and arterial highways almost automatically calls forth a certain volume of federal expenditures, region by region. Many of these expenditures serve regional needs for government services in exactly the same way that they are served by state or local governments. Programs for national recreation areas, public housing, veterans hospitals, and urban renewal are programs in point. As an accounting matter, federal programs that are implemented by grants-in-aid are now reflected in state- and local-government accounts. What is needed is to deal directly with federal goods and services transactions and to include these in a regional governments account.

If a case can be made for treating federal-government activity within a region as "regional government," then, of course, an even stronger case can be made for assigning state-government activities to regions. State-government programs are now, and will increasingly be, directed toward metropolitan areas. If these are the regions of primary concern, state-government programs for health and hospitals, streets and highways, higher education, and recreation are substitutes for and supplements to local-government programs. All of this suggests that there are really no very formidable conceptual obstacles in assigning federal and state expenditures to local areas and in consolidating the expenditures of federal, state, and local governments into a single regional governments account.

There are, however, some serious obstacles on the revenue side. For expenditures it is proposed that national, state, and local outlays all be viewed as benefiting the residents of the region in which the expenditures are made. Spillover benefits are to be neglected. A corollary approach to revenue would require that all federal, state, and local taxes whose incidence falls on the region should be recorded on the revenue side of the regional governments account. This approach would permit the estimation of a regional government fiscal residuum to reveal the net primary fiscal advantage that a region obtained as a result of the revenue-expenditure impact of the national and state governments.

This approach, however, requires more knowledge of the incidence of taxes than is now possessed by public-finance economists. A cursory reading of contemporary literature on incidence theory suggests that at the moment there is considerable disenchantment with the traditional partial-equilibrium approach to incidence and a recognition that some kind of general-equilibrium analysis is required.[21] But the theoretical underpinnings are now so weak that it is difficult to undertake the necessary empirical work. The recent Labovitz study allocates federal activity by states; the Musgrave-Daicoff study estimates Michigan state- and local-tax burdens on Michigan residents; the Brownlee study estimates state-tax and -expenditure benefits for Minnesota.[22] But there are no studies that embrace all government activity or even all government revenue for a specific region.

Some value would, of course, attach to a regional-government-revenue account that simply recorded collections, and data of this kind are available. A collection basis would record federal cigarette taxes at the cigarette factories in North Carolina and Virginia. It would record personal income taxes in the region of domicile rather than in the region where the taxpayer worked and earned his income, for those who commute or receive income across regional lines. It would record corporate-profits taxes in the region where the headquarters is located, as Leven proposed, in the absence of a better solution, for the regional attribution of corporate profits.[23] A possible but not wholly satisfactory alternative for the corporate-profits tax would be to assign the levy to specific regions on the basis of the traditional Massachusetts formula used for the allocation of corporate net income for state-tax purposes. This formula utilizes an average of three measures—sales, wages and salaries paid, and the book value of property.

Aside from this tax-type solution for corporate-profits taxes there would appear to be no intermediate choice. Either the regional-government-revenue account records collections or it records estimated burdens, where such estimates reflect a host of arbitrary assumptions about the spatial incidence of all the taxes in the tax system. Nevertheless, the choice is clearly in favor of

[21] See, for example, A. R. Prest, *Public Finance* (Chicago: Quadrangle Books, 1960), pp. 30–90.

[22] I. M. Labovitz, *Federal Revenues and Expenditures in the Several States* (Washington: Legislative Reference Service, Library of Congress, 1962); Richard A. Musgrave and Darwin W. Daicoff, "Who Pays Michigan Taxes?," *Staff Papers* (Lansing: Michigan Tax Study, 1958), pp. 131–51; O. H. Brownlee, *Estimated Distribution of Minnesota Taxes and Public Expenditure Benefits* (Minneapolis: University of Minnesota Press, 1960).

[23] Charles L. Leven, in Hochwald, *op. cit.*, p. 160.

the latter approach, in spite of the unresolved problems. Collection data are not particularly meaningful for the analysis of government activities. Even the arbitrary assignment of federal and state taxes to regions on the basis of population or income would be preferable to collections data alone.

Apart from the problems on the revenue side, there are some difficulties in a regional governments account that are occasioned by the multiplicity of local-government units. School districts, water districts, fire districts, and transportation districts have boundaries that are not coterminous with those of municipalities or even of counties. In consequence, there is the practical task of assigning the activities of these districts to appropriate municipalities. Sacks and Carroll have demonstrated that this can be done in New York State, where the special-district problem is about as serious as anywhere. They have succeeded in assigning all local-government activity, including that involved in school districts, to the municipalities served by the districts.[24] However, the unavailability of data may make this arrangement almost impossible in other states.

Both these matters—the assignment of federal- and state-government revenue to regions, and the treatment of the multiplicity of local governments—would be greatly eased if one were interested only in a consolidated regional governments account for an area at least as large as a Standard Metropolitan Statistical Area, and not in spatial disaggregation below that level. This, however, should not be the objective. If a regional government account is to have maximum usefulness, it should be built up from data for constituent municipalities. Municipalities are major decision units for government activity within a region. If a government account is to serve useful policy purposes—these to be described in a moment —disaggregation should be carried to the municipal level.

A remaining general problem in the classification of government activity in the region is the treatment of non-profit organizations. The dividing line between private and public economic activity is rather sharper in this country than in a great many other coun-

[24] Seymour Sacks and John Carroll, *Revenues, Expenditures and Debt: 1949–1959* (Albany: New York State Department of Audit and Control, 1961).

tries. There are relatively few of the mixed-enterprise operations so characteristic of the industrial, financial, and development undertakings of both Western European and South American countries. Nevertheless, classification difficulties are posed by a number of non-profit activities, particularly in health, welfare, and recreation.

Private hospitals are substitutes for government hospitals; private recreation programs are substitutes for public recreation programs; the Community Chest is more public than private in most communities. Obviously, it would be convenient to put all such activities into the private sector, but if a regional governments account is to show something about program levels such semipublic activities should, in some fashion, be taken into account. Perhaps this could be accomplished by an information statement on public activity, with governmental and semigovernmental activities as sub-categories. The criterion for the semigovernmental activities might rest on some rough concept of opportunity cost: if the private activity were not in existence, would government be required to assume the program responsibility?

Finally, it may be noted that any classification of regional government must embrace all forms in which government activity is conducted. These are traditionally three: public enterprise, trust funds, and general government. There are some difficult accounting problems in consolidating these diverse types of activities, but it would surely be inappropriate to resolve these difficulties by combining public enterprise with the private sector. Ideally, subsidiary accounts should permit distinctions among the three types of government organization since the decision patterns that affect them are substantially different.

3. THE PURPOSES TO BE SERVED

In this examination of purposes no effort will be made to distinguish the data necessary for the measurement of government activity in prior periods from the data necessary for projection. It will be assumed, and surely this is not open to debate, that projections, and public and private decisions based on such projections, will be more realistic and "better" if grounded on the best available data descriptive of prior-period government activity.

Perhaps the most important policy purpose to be served by a comprehensive set of regional governments accounts is the provision of data relevant for the planning and construction of public facilities.

The definition of government capital for regional purposes poses no particular difficulty in the case of state and local governments. A great many such governments have a capital budget, with a definition of capital closely tied to traditional public-works concepts based on life expectancy. One-year or three-year cut-offs are used to distinguish capital from operating expenditures. But the definition of federal-government capital for regional purposes raises all the age-old questions that have been controverted and unanswered for many years. Are expenditures for military installations properly classified as current or capital? What about arterial highways? National monuments? In recent years, as a result of work in development economics plus the rediscovery of the investment character of education, there has been a tendency to think increasingly of a number of government programs, formerly classified as current, as truly capital in nature.

No effort will be made here to struggle again with the definitional problems inherent in this hardy perennial. For purposes of establishing a regional governments account to embrace national-government capital expenditures it would be highly desirable to be as conservative as possible, to narrow the definition of federal-government capital and to keep this definition close to the public-works concept: let it consist of hospitals, arterial highways, water-resource investment—in short, physical facilities probably both military and non-military.

Government capital expenditures must be classified by function, that is, in such broad program categories as public safety, highways, water, sewerage, education, welfare, and health (see Appendix A). The functional classification generally tends to follow department and agency lines, particularly for state and local governments, and thus conforms with traditional budget classification. The consolidated regional governments capital account would then aggregate the separate capital accounts of the federal, state, and local governments within the region. The capital expenditures of public enterprise should likewise be reflected in the consolidated account.

There are, of course, capital revenues to be matched against capital expenditures. The proceeds of borrowing by state and local governments, although not technically a capital revenue, should be identified. Depreciation allowances are available for financing the capital expenditures of public undertakings, although general government agencies do not, of course, maintain depreciation accounts.

In addition to the regional-government capital account prepared annually, periodic subsidiary information statements are very much needed. As noted above, such statements could report the capital outlays of semipublic agencies. And in the public sector supplementary information is needed on the age, condition, life expectancy, and technological usefulness of existing stocks of facilities. All such characteristics unfortunately have spatial dimensions as well as physical and technological ones. The existence of unused capacity in the water system in one part of the region will not obviate the need for building additional facilities elsewhere in the region. A complete inventory will require some mapping.

A regional governments capital account along the foregoing lines could be expected to be useful in a number of ways. It will not, of course, be used for central regionwide decisions about government capital facilities; governments are too fragmented for that. But the account should in itself encourage attention to intergovernmental planning relationships within the region. It may even encourage the extension of capital budgeting techniques to local governments that do not now employ this device. These are modest goals but worthy ones.

In a well-articulated procedure for capital-facilities planning in local government, the projection of physical requirements precedes the preparation of the long-range financial plan for physical facilities —the capital budget projection, as it is usually termed. Financial possibilities—for grants-in-aid, for bond financing, for service charges —will of course modify, as they should, decisions about the physical facilities that are planned for construction. Decisions about capital facilities are not made solely in relation to need or in relation to efficiency in the conduct of the public sector, but in relation, in part, to the availability of funds. A comprehensive regional-government capital account will not change this framework; it should, however, make it more orderly.

The second purpose to be served by the regional governments accounts is in long-range fiscal planning. Fiscal planning requires a capital account, to be sure, but beyond this it requires a carefully constructed current account. On the expenditure side, the current account should again be functionalized with the same classification as for the capital account. The distinction between goods and services outlays and transfer payments is, of course, important in analyzing the income-generating effects of government activity but is much less significant for general fiscal purposes.

The important information that is needed and that is so often lacking now on a regional basis is a breakdown of sources of revenue. The local-government revenue account for each constituent municipal area should distinguish grants-in-aid and shared taxes from locally imposed levies. This is conventional enough, but the serious weakness in existing revenue accounts is inadequacy of data on the property tax. This kind of information can probably best be presented in subsidiary statements, but as things now stand any analysis of the behavior of the property tax is greatly handicapped by the absence of information on revenues by class of property (residential, industrial, commercial, etc.), and on the extent to which increases in property-tax revenue are attributable to new construction, to changes in assessments on existing property, and to rate increases. The compilation of such data for each municipal area and its aggregation into a local-government account for the region would permit a more accurate appraisal of the fiscal position of local government vis-à-vis the state and federal governments. Local-government fiscal capacity is so closely linked with the property tax that projection of its fiscal future requires the maximum of useful data.

A regional governments account would more effectively serve up the data necessary for projection of both revenue and expenditure than an account that is restricted solely to local government within a region. A projection model using multiple regression techniques, such as that developed by Hirsch for St. Louis County, could then utilize, as dependent variables, per-capita expenditures of all governments for specified functions, rather than expenditures of local governments alone.[25]

An integrated current and capital account for all governments within a region would provide the prerequisite information for analyzing the levels and effectiveness of governmental programs. This could be the beginning of the efforts that must be made to quantify levels of government services, over time and among municipalities and regions.[26] An integrated set of accounts should also have as a by-product an encouragement to local-government officials to examine their capital and operating programs in relationship one to the other.

A third purpose may eventually be served by a consolidated regional governments account. It may be possible in the not too distant future to translate levels of government activity, and in particular government capital-facilities programs, into estimated land-use requirements.[27] Such requirements could then be projected in physical terms at specified locations within a region and controlled by land-use planning, zoning, and subdivision regulations. In some metropolitan areas certain kinds of public land-use requirements, as for recreation, are now partially planned and controlled, although requirements are typically projected solely as a function of population. The suggestion here is that land-use projections could be refined and made more realistic through explicit linkage with government revenue and expenditure data in a regional governments account. We will probably never reach a high degree of refinement in any projections of land-use requirements, but the assignment is so important to the future of urban economic development that almost any modest contribution in this direction will be useful.[28]

[25] Werner Z. Hirsch, in Bollens, *op. cit.*, pp. 353–68, 388–403, 453–57.
[26] See Hirsch, "Quality of Government Services," in Howard G. Schaller (ed.), *Public Expenditure Decisions in the Urban Community*, papers presented at a conference sponsored by the Committee on Urban Economics, May 14–15, 1962 (Washington: Resources for the Future, Inc., 1963).
[27] See Lloyd Rodwin, "Metropolitan Policy for Developing Areas," in Isard and Cumberland, *op. cit.*, pp. 227–28.
[28] Richard B. Andrews, "Urban Economics: An Appraisal of Progress," *Land Economics*, August 1961, p. 223.

4. REGIONAL ACCOUNTS AND REGIONAL DECISIONS

A regional governments account and the supporting schedules suggested here would go far to meet the data requirements suggested by Harvey Perloff in his preliminary draft memorandum, "The Public and Household Sectors in Regional Accounts" (April 1961), and elaborated further in the Perloff-Leven paper appearing later in this volume. Government expenditures within the region would be classified by function, by level of government (federal, state, local), and by form of government organization, with distinctions between capital and operating expenditures and between goods and services payments and transfer payments. Expenditures so classified could then be arrayed against the subject or clientele population served. As noted, these steps would constitute the beginnings of an attempt to measure government-service levels. Expenditure accounts of this nature are not, of course, a substitute for the traditional object accounting that is used by all governments for purposes of financial control. The accounts proposed here are supplementary to existing accounting techniques.

A regional governments account, particularly if co-ordinated with an information matrix along the Perloff-Leven lines, should contribute substantially to an improved flow of information for public decisions. We would be farther ahead if government expenditures in the region could be divided between autonomous and derived.

The distinction is this: some government activities within a region are a function of the economic-activity levels of households and business firms. Let this portion of government expenditures be classified as derived. There is another portion of government activity in the region that is autonomous, that is, independent of the activity levels of households and business firms. In an input-output framework, making this distinction amounts to shifting a part of government activity into the processing sector with an equivalent reduction of that portion of government that is treated as final demand.[29] This implies the existence of production coefficients for the portion of government activity in the processing sector.

[29] Charles L. Leven, in Hochwald, *op. cit.*, pp. 183–84.

For example, a very large part of the local-government services associated with middle-income residential development may be classified as derived. A suburban residential development with households of specified characteristics with respect to income, age, occupation, and ethnic status will be accompanied by a volume of government activity that probably varies within rather narrow limits. Such residential developments give rise to a governmental package of public education, streets and roads, police and fire protection, water supply, and sewage disposal. Decision patterns within municipalities and other local-government units respond in a highly predictable fashion to provide this package. Some programs of state governments, particularly established grant-in-aid arrangements, likewise exhibit a smooth response to local area characteristics. Some federal-government activities are similarly derived from the level and composition of local economic activity—again, the operations of the Post Office Department are an example.

On the other hand, there are a great many governmental activities—federal, state, and local—that ought to be classified as autonomous with respect to the region. These are programs whose levels or volume of activity are not easily explainable as derivative of the measurable characteristics of households and business firms. A New Haven makes a massive breakthrough in urban renewal; a Syracuse initiates a water-supply program to take care of regional needs for several decades. The forces that give rise to such "autonomous" government programs consist of complex social, economic, and political phenomena that now elude our ability to quantify.

Our present understanding of the determinants of the demand for and the supply of governmental services at the regional level probably does not permit a classification system or a set of regional governments accounts based on the distinction between autonomous and derived as suggested here. But it is suggested here that the distinction is important and exists in the world reflected in government budgets. As we come to understand better the measurable characteristics of urbanization that are associated with the measurable characteristics of regional public finances, it may be possible to incorporate this significant distinction into a system of accounts.

APPENDIX A

The Regional Governments Account (Simplified Accounts)

	Local and special districts			State			Federal			Total		
	1	2	3	4	5	6	7	8	9	10	11	12
	Region	Rest of world	Total	Region	Rest of world	Total	Region	Rest of world	Total	Region	Rest of world	Total
I. General Government Current Account												
A. Expenditure												
1. National security °												
2. International affairs °												
3. Veterans												
4. Commerce and labor												
5. Agriculture												
6. Other natural resources												
7. Housing and community redevelopment												
8. Public safety												
9. Highways												
10. Education												
11. Libraries												
12. Public welfare												
13. Health and hospitals												
14. Water												
15. Sewerage												
16. General control												
17. Interest												
18. Other												
Total °												
B. Revenue °												
1. Income taxes on individuals												
2. Corporate income and capital stock taxes												
3. General sales taxes												
4. Other excises												
5. Customs												
6. Property taxes												
7. Estate and gift												
8. Other												
Total												
C. Surplus or deficit on current account (A − B)												
II. General Government Capital Account												
A. Expenditure												
1. National security °												

° See Appendix B: Notes.

	Local and special districts			State			Federal			Total		
	1	2	3	4	5	6	7	8	9	10	11	12
	Region	Rest of world	Total	Region	Rest of world	Total	Region	Rest of world	Total	Region	Rest of world	Total
2. International affairs °												
3. Veterans												
4. Commerce and labor												
5. Agriculture												
6. Other natural resources												
7. Housing and community redevelopment												
8. Public safety												
9. Highways												
10. Education												
11. Libraries												
12. Public welfare												
13. Health and hospitals												
14. Water												
15. Sewerage												
16. General control												
18. Other												
Total °												
B. Revenue												
1. Sales of assets												
2. Repayment of loans												
3. Transfers from current revenue												
4. Proceeds of borrowing °												
Total												
C. Surplus or deficit on capital account (A − B)												
III. Public Enterprise Current Account †												
A. Expenditure												
1. Wages and salaries												
2. Other goods and services												
3. Interest												
4. Tax payments												
5. Depreciation allowances												
6. Decrease (−) or increase (+) in inventories of purchased goods												
Total												

° See Appendix B: Notes.
† Identified by functional categories 1–16, 18 (I-A).

APPENDIX A *(Continued)*
The Regional Governments Account (Simplified Accounts)

	Local and special districts			State			Federal			Total		
	1	2	3	4	5	6	7	8	9	10	11	12
	Region	Rest of world	Total	Region	Rest of world	Total	Region	Rest of world	Total	Rest of world	Region	Total

B. Revenue
  1. Sales of goods and services
  2. Interest and dividends
  3. Increase (+) or decrease (−) in inventories of goods in process

    Total

C. Surplus or deficit on current account (A − B)

IV. Public Enterprise Capital Account †

A. Expenditure
  1. Buildings and other construction
  2. Machinery and equipment
  3. Additions to inventory

    Total: gross capital formation

  4. Purchase or redemption of own obligations
  5. Purchase of obligations issued by others

    Total: expenditures

B. Revenue
  1. Depreciation allowances
  2. Sales of own obligations
  3. Sales of obligations issued by others
  4. Repayment of obligations issued by others
  5. Decreases in inventory

    Total

C. Surplus or deficit on capital account (A − B)

† Identified by functional categories 1–16, 18 (I-A).

	Local and special districts			State			Federal			Total		
	1	2	3	4	5	6	7	8	9	10	11	12
	Region	Rest of world	Total	Region	Rest of world	Total	Region	Rest of world	Total	Region	Rest of world	Total
V. Trust Fund Current Account [*]												
A. Expenditure												
1. Administrative expenses												
2. Transfers or payments to beneficiaries												
Total												
B. Revenue												
1. Employer taxes												
2. Employee taxes												
3. Interest												
Total												
C. Surplus or deficit on current account (A − B)												

	1 General Govt. Capital	2 General Govt. Current	3 Pub. Ent. Capital	4 Pub. Ent. Current	5 Trust Funds	6 Total
VI. Consolidated Account: Regional Transactions (from Column 10)						
A. Expenditure (All items)	(I-A)	(II-A)	(III-A)	(IV-A)	(V-A)	
Total						
B. Revenue (All items)	(I-B) [*]	(II-B)	(III-B)	(IV-B)	(V-B)	
Total						
C. Net total surplus or deficit on transactions account [*]	(A-B)					
VII. Consolidated Account: Regional Programs (from Column 12)						
A. Expenditure (All items)	(I-A)	(II-A)	(III-A)	(IV-A)	(V-A)	
Total						
B. Revenue (All items)	(I-B)	(II-B)	(III-B)	(IV-B)	(V-B)	
Total						
C. Fiscal residuum on program account (A − B)						

[*] See Appendix B: Notes.

APPENDIX B: NOTES

The Simplified Accounts are constructed on the assumption that two kinds of financial information are needed for a regional governments account: (1) expenditures and revenues for governments within the region where such revenue-expenditure transactions subtract from or add to private-sector incomes within the region (this is the information necessary for input-output); and (2) expenditure-revenue information that will reveal program levels within the region.

The latter requires that the distinction between region and rest of world be carried through the expenditure accounts, and through all revenue accounts except for general government current revenue. In this case all revenue for local and special districts will presumably be collected from firms and households in the region and shifting to outsiders may be neglected. State and local current revenue on general government accounts for the region must be estimated in accordance with the presumed regional burden of state and federal taxes.

The necessity for the distinction between (1) and (2) may be illustrated by reference to library expenditures. A local library purchases books outside the region. Such a purchase does not add to regional income, but it must be counted in the library's program outlays if service levels are to be measured.

Ideally, the degree of refinement illustrated here should be carried through for each municipal area, but in practice it may be necessary to aggregate for the region as a whole.

I-A, 1-2; II-A, 1-2. An attempt to measure regional-program levels as a reflection of both in-region and out-of-region expenditures is conceptually awkward in the case of national security and international affairs. Such a treatment would imply that regional-program levels (benefits) can be measured as separable components of national programs, an implication that ought to be rejected. Therefore, the rest-of-world breakdown should be omitted on these two lines, for both the current and capital accounts.

I-A (Total). These totals may be subject to further classification in additional memorandum accounts, to distinguish, for example, between goods and services transactions and transfer payments.

I-B, VI-B (Column 1). No in-region breakdown is used for the general government current-revenue account; the totals must therefore be entered in VI-B, Column 1.

II-A (Total). These totals may be further classified, if interest attaches to the distinction, into new construction, producer durables, additions to inventory, and purchases of existing assets.

V. It is assumed that trust funds have no capital account except for financial transactions.

VI-C. Net total surplus or deficit on transactions account should equal government final demand in a regional interindustry matrix less tax payments of regional households and firms to government. Therefore, if transfer payments are excluded from final demand, they must correspondingly be excluded from the expenditure totals in VI-A.

COMMENT

HARVEY E. BRAZER
U.S. Treasury Department

Given the assignment of a difficult topic, Professor Burkhead has produced a paper which covers the subject most effectively. I find only a few points with which I should like to take issue or upon which some comment is called for.

Is there really, as Burkhead maintains in agreement with Clark Bloom, "no compelling problem that dominates the field of regional analysis to give it focus in the same way that economic stabilization has dominated macroeconomics and the monopoly problem has dominated microeconomics"? It seems to me that regional analysis and location theory are inseparable and that the location of economic activity does give rise not to one but to a multitude of "compelling problems." A policy orientation is surely suggested by our concern with such problems as are involved in the movement of industry from central cities to suburbs and the movement of industries such as the textile and automobile industries from one region of the country to another, the specter of depressed areas, and the human and economic problems related to unemployment and underemployment in many of the rural areas of the nation. I should look to regional analysis to provide policy insights that may be useful for guidance purposes with respect to the programs of the Area Redevelopment Administration, state and local efforts to woo industry, etc.

It is true that every region contains its multiplicity of government units, often working at cross-purposes and in conflict with one another, but this is not to suggest, as Burkhead seems to imply, that we can do nothing but throw up our hands in frustration. Rather, we need to seek, partly through regional analysis, as much knowledge as can be obtained about the framework of operation of these governmental units, and we should make every effort to develop the insights that will enable us, at a minimum, to count the costs of the absence of co-ordination.

Perhaps Burkhead puts his finger on the problem of the inadequacy of regional analysis when he points out that "Accounting structures are not equipped to handle such variables [extraregional forces such as national policy, changes in technology, political power structure of a region], particularly in an open economy." What this suggests, of course, is that regional analysis must go further than the distance involved in merely developing accounting structures. If it stops at that point it is indeed unlikely to prove very fruitful.

Burkhead properly emphasizes the need to trace the regional economic-process effects of national and state expenditures and the regional incidence of national and state as well as local taxes. I should hope, however, that as economists we might do better than to follow his suggestion, in the case of the corporate-profits tax, that the tax be assigned on the basis of the so-called Massachusetts allocation formula. I see no rational reason for allocation on the basis of an average of sales, wages and salaries paid, and the value of property. Application of this formula suggests that each of the three factors should carry equal weight. But it seems clear to me that the sales factor may be irrelevant, or nearly so, and that allocation on the basis of the location of economic inputs, particularly the input of capital, makes much better economic sense. I am not at all sure, however, that regional incidence is always more relevant than regional impact. Perhaps in the case of the local property tax, for example, we should revert to the English neoclassical distinction between "onerous" and "beneficial" levies. The latter are essentially in the nature of user charges and may be regarded as prices paid for economic inputs in the form of government services. The former, on the other hand, are of quite a different order and cannot readily be treated within the same framework of analysis for regional accounting purposes.

I cannot agree with Burkhead's suggestion that "Perhaps the most important policy purpose to be served by a comprehensive set of regional governments accounts is the provision of data relevant for the planning and construction of public facilities." This is certainly an important policy purpose, but surely it is only one of many that are at least equally important. Others that suggest themselves are the allocation of costs among governmental units within a region of joint ventures in the provision of public services, the definition of those services that should be provided on a regional basis, the measurement of spillover effects, etc.

Toward the end of his paper Burkhead makes the point that I should have thought central to the paper as a whole—that is, that a regional governments account "should contribute substantially to an improved flow of information for public decisions." But I cannot share his view that there is anything to be gained from dividing government expenditures within a region between "autonomous" and "derived" expenditures. He suggests that derived expenditures are those which are a function of the levels of economic activity of households and business firms, whereas autonomous expenditures are independent of such levels of economic activity. This suggestion, it seems to me, implies far too narrow a definition of the factors contributing to the demand for government services or expenditures. I should argue that the demand for government expenditures is "derived" from a variety of forces, of which levels of economic activity of households and business in a region constitute but one set. In fact Burkhead is somewhat inconsistent or unclear on this subject, since he first suggests that derived expenditures are given by levels of economic activity and then argues that "A suburban residential development with households of specified characteristics with respect to income, age, occupation, and ethnic status will be accompanied by a volume of government activity that probably varies within rather narrow limits." If to these factors one adds religious and political preference there seems no reason to exclude from consideration the forces that Burkhead suggests determine "autonomous" government expenditures in the form of "complex social, economic, and political phenomena that now elude our ability to quantify." The fact that a variable is not amenable to quantification does not necessarily exclude it from analysis of the forces determining the levels and directions of government expenditures. The so-called "dummy" variable is a very useful device for application where a given social or economic characteristic is not quantifiable.[1] Clearly I prefer to avoid a distinction between different kinds of government expenditures that is based on our present ability to "explain" variations in their levels among communities. It may be going too far to suggest that there is no such thing as "autonomous" expenditures in the sense in which Burkhead uses the term. But until a great deal more work has been done in this area I should deplore the implied suggestion that the unknown is unknowable or that the unexplained is inexplicable.

COMMENT

KARL A. FOX
Iowa State University

This is not so much a comment as a lay sermon for which Jesse Burkhead's opening sentences supply the text:

Those who have worked in recent years at the development of regional concepts and at the measurement of regional economic activity are by this time aware that their efforts have no clear-cut policy orientation. Regional accounting is not directed toward a set of regional policies nor toward an organizational structure, public or private, with responsibility for regional well-being. The meas-

[1] For a recent illustration of the use of dummy variables, see Harvey E. Brazer, Daniel B. Suits, and Muriel W. Converse, "Municipal Bond Yields: The Market's Reaction to Michigan's Fiscal Crisis," *National Tax Journal*, March 1962, pp. 66–70.

urement of levels of private economic activity within a region does not in any sense imply, for example, that there is or should be a regional trade policy or a regional development policy, a point which was well made by Werner Hochwald in his 1957 paper. And, as Clark Bloom pointed out in his review of Isard's *Methods of Regional Analysis*, there is no compelling problem that dominates the field of regional analysis to give it focus in the same way that economic stabilization has dominated macroeconomics, and the monopoly problem has dominated microeconomics.[1]

These statements are indeed applicable to much recent and current work in regional accounting. But as I have pointed out on other occasions, it is possible to delineate a set of regions which will provide a compelling problem and a policy orientation for regional accounts. Given an appropriate region, a rigorous logical framework is available for stating and analyzing the corresponding set of policy problems.

A very important literature on the theory of economic policy has developed in the last few years, and it seems to me that it has been generally ignored by regional economists. It has been ignored partly because (1) there has been no consensus as to the size and type of region for which accounts should be kept and (2) so long as the type of region is unspecified, the nature of the associated policy problems remains obscure. However, once we have defined a policy-oriented region and the class of problems appropriate to it, we have good reason for seeking improvements in the policy-making process.

Jan Tinbergen made a major breakthrough in the analysis of economic policies in a series of books published from 1952 to 1956.[2] Further extensions and applications have been made by Theil,[3] Van Eijk and Sandee,[4] and others. Tinbergen was primarily con-

[1] See Burkhead paper, above.

[2] Jan Tinbergen, *On the Theory of Economic Policy; Centralization and Decentralization in Economic Policy;* and *Economic Policy: Principles and Design* (Amsterdam: North-Holland Publishing Co., 1952, 1954, and 1956, respectively).

[3] H. Theil, "On the Theory of Economic Policy," *American Economic Review,* 45 (May 1956), 360–66; and *Economic Forecasts and Policy,* 2d rev. ed. (Amsterdam: North-Holland Publishing Co., 1961).

[4] C. J. Van Eijk and J. Sandee, "Quantitative Determination of an Optimum Economic Policy," *Econometrica,* 27 (Jan. 1959), 1–13.

cerned with the development of consistent economic policies at the national level. However, his model can readily be adapted to smaller areas and political jurisdictions.

To illustrate Tinbergen's framework, let us assume that we are looking at the United States economy from the viewpoint, say, of a chairman of the Council of Economic Advisers. Our first requirement is an accurate knowledge of the workings of the economy. Certain variables will generally constitute the targets or goals of economic policy—the level of employment, the price level, the level of real income per capita, the distribution of income, the balance of payments, and perhaps others. Assume for the moment that values have been specified for each of the target variables for the coming year: let us simply say that they are targets the President would like to see the economy achieve (presumably after listening to advice from many people).

The actual performance of the economy will depend upon two sorts of factors. First, there are a number of variables which are not controllable by the government of the United States; the best we can hope to do is to forecast the values they will assume during the year ahead. If we also know the net effect of a unit change in each of the non-controllable factors upon each of the target variables, we can forecast (with greater or less accuracy) the levels that each of the target variables will likely attain if there is no change in present economic policies.

If we are lucky enough to find the various sectors of the economy moving in the right directions at the right speeds, all the goals may be achieved without special effort. However, the government has at its disposal an array of policy instruments that can be used to influence the target variables in the desired direction if it appears that the non-controllable factors (or "data," as Tinbergen calls them) will not do the job. These instruments include all the actions legally permitted to the federal government and its agencies which would have some effect on the course of the economy.

To use these instruments with confidence, the policy-maker (or at least the adviser) should know the net effect of a unit change in each instrument upon each of the goals or target variables. In addition, use of the policy instruments will have side effects on other economic variables; however, we may decide that these are not sufficiently important to warrant concern. These last variables, which Tinbergen refers to as "irrelevant" with respect to a given problem, are also affected by the "data" or non-controllable factors.

The basic technical problem is to determine with sufficient accuracy the system of structural relations which connects all the variables and which constitutes a model of the economy. This model will include, among other variables, major components of the national income and product accounts. Given an adequate model, the problem of economic policy is to use instruments in such a way that the specified goals are achieved in spite of disturbances arising from the non-controllable factors.

Let us examine Tinbergen's approach more closely. First, all the variables in his scheme are measurable economic magnitudes. They are related by a system of simultaneous equations. The variables are divided into two categories, *exogenous* and *endogenous*. Effects run *from* the exogenous *to* the endogenous variables within the time unit for which the model is designed (usually a year, although the newer econometric models of the United States are based on quarterly data). The equation system is designed to answer the following questions: (1) Given a set of known or projected values of the exogenous variables for the coming year, what values of the endogenous variables are likely to emerge? (2) Given desired values of the target variables and forecasts of the non-controllable factors, what "settings" of the policy instruments are required to achieve the target values?

The second major element in Tinbergen's approach is introduced not by the economist but by the policy-maker. In principle, the model of the economy is objective, reproducible, and non-political —"value-free." In Tinbergen's scheme, the policy-maker is responsible for classifying the endogenous variables into those which have significant effects on welfare (target variables) and those which have negligible effects (irrelevant variables). He may judge also that a unit increase in one target contributes three times as much to welfare as a unit increase in a second target but only half as much as a unit increase in a third. He classifies the exogenous variables into non-controllable factors and potential instruments. For the most part, changes in both categories affect welfare through their influence upon the target variables. However, the policy-maker may decide that the use of certain instruments involves direct welfare losses which must be offset against the welfare gains resulting from their effects upon the target variables.

Different policy-makers would assign different value weights to the same target. Given the same facts about the structure of the economy and its current position, one might be willing to accept a 3-per-cent rise in prices to achieve a 1-per-cent increase in employment, while another might be willing to accept only a 1-per-cent price rise for the same employment gain. The two policy-makers have different marginal rates of substitution between these goals—different value systems or "welfare functions."

It seems to me that Tinbergen's approach can also be applied to the policy problems of a state or smaller political jurisdiction. (Bear in mind that the Functional Economic Area could become a political jurisdiction if state and national leaders wished this to be so.) In any given year, legislation and policies of the federal government would be "data" or non-controllable factors for the state. The array of policy instruments available to the governor would differ from the array available to the President. Also, in assigning weights to the various policy targets subject to his influence, the governor would be responsible to the people of the state rather than to those of the entire nation. In general, side effects upon residents of other states would be disregarded, and events in other states would be non-controllable factors. Targets and instruments would be related through a model of the economy of the state.

Obviously, we can apply this approach to the policy problems confronting a mayor, a city council, or a county board of supervisors. Actions of the state government must now be taken as "data"; the model needed now relates to the economy of a town or county; and actions of governments, consumers, or businessmen in other towns and counties within the state also affect the ease or difficulty with which the local officials can achieve their goals.

As readily as to government policy-making the scheme can be adapted to the policy problems of voluntary groups which are trying to improve the economy of a functional economic area that cuts across county lines. The voluntary group may be able to influence directly only a few aspects of the area economy; yet it needs to know enough about the complete structure of the economy to estimate the indirect effects of its proposed actions.

The significance of Tinbergen's approach in relation to the application of regional accounts to functional economic areas is simply this: It shows how detailed information about the structure of the area's economy can be explicitly incorporated into the design of development and other policies for the area. At the same time, it enables us to separate questions of fact about economic relationships from questions of value about community goals and the acceptability of alternative means for achieving them.

DATA FOR THE PUBLIC-FINANCE SUB-ACCOUNT

DICK NETZER

Graduate School of Public Administration,
New York University, and Regional Plan Association
(New York)

In his successful effort to make public finance and regional economics say something meaningful to one another within the framework of regional accounts, Jesse Burkhead has indicated the magnitude of the demands for data and also suggested some of the obstacles to satisfying these demands. The lack of policy orientation in regional accounts, the paucity of quite ordinary data on the government sector, the rather sketchy treatment of the sector in regional-accounts development heretofore, and the need for a family of subsidiary statements not easily integrated into the frameworks of over-all regional-economic-activity accounts generate challenges and problems for both conceptual-development and statistical-development work. In regard to the latter, to use Burkhead's collection of adjectives (applied to another research problem), the problems are opaque, thorny, and a mare's nest and the raw material is obscure, ineluctable, elusive, and intractable.

In view of this appraisal, the present effort has limited objectives: to discuss the kinds of data needed for alternative treatments of the government sector in regional accounts, especially that developed in Burkhead's paper; to identify the gaps and appraise their seriousness; and to suggest, in some cases, what might be done to improve matters.

1. THE SHORTCOMINGS OF AVAILABLE DATA

As Burkhead has indicated, the government sector typically has been given short shrift in regional-accounting frameworks, whether input-output models, income and product accounts, or balance-of-payments statements.[1] Local government has been suppressed into the household sector and government has been treated as an intermediate product, so that it has been denied any autonomous role; relations with "outside" governments have been treated in a mechanical and quite artificial manner, also seriously affecting the operational qualities of the models for purposes of public policy. Given the specific objectives of the account builders in these instances, or rather, of their sponsors, the marginal efficiency of investing their limited resources in intellectually more satisfying treatment of the government sector in preference to the many alternative claims obviously was not encouraging, although the temper of the times—the mid-1950's—surely affected the weights used in making the choice. Nevertheless, the treatments employed, despite their conceptual abbreviation, were not easy ways out of the data problem.

Take, for example, Leven's set of accounts, as applied to Sioux City, Iowa.[2] Here the goal, as I understand it, was to identify the exogenous forces operating in the Sioux City economy and in the framework of income and product accounting to project not only income but also employment, population, and land requirements for a sponsor concerned with both capital budgeting and land-use controls. As Burkhead noted, the local-government sector is largely suppressed in this arrangement; non-local governments are hardly treated exhaustively, either. Despite this, consider the list of data requirements for the base year (1958):[3]

---

[1] See Burkhead's references to Artle; Hochwald, Striner, and Sonenblum; Leven; and Berman, Chinitz, and Hoover, for example. Also, Federal Reserve Bank of Chicago, *Methods and Sources for Estimates of the Balance of Payments of a Metropolitan Area* (April 1957); Sioux City, Iowa, City Planning Commission, *Economic Report 1959*.

[2] In Sioux City Planning Commission, *op. cit.*

[3] Obviously, for projections, one should not be satisfied with coefficients for a *single* base year, a fact that further complicated the data problem.

Tax and non-tax payments from the area's residents and businesses to state and federal governments, classified by
>   indirect business taxes
>   corporate-income-tax liability
>   employment taxes
>   personal-income-tax liability

Transfer payments from state and federal governments to the area's businesses, residents, and local governments.

State- and federal-government payrolls in the area (and, in concept at least, remittances "abroad" by the recipients of these payrolls).

Capital formation by all levels of government in the area.

Imports of final and intermediate goods for government-capital formation.

Local-government "consumption" expenditures.

Imports of final and intermediate goods for local-government "consumption" expenditures.

Receipts of interest on debt of governments outside the area by local residents and organizations.

Payments of interest on debt of area governments to holders located outside the area.

There is not a single item in the list for which data are readily at hand. Census data provide some of the needed material on local-government finances, but in detail and on a metropolitan-area-wide basis only for quinquennial Census years. Financial reports of state and local governments provide some supplementary detail, including, for some taxes and transfers and some forms of state-government direct expenditure, data on state programs by county and/or by municipality. Household surveys conducted in the course of such studies provide some data on the household sector's relations with government. But after all these fragments are pieced together most of the cells are still empty and must be filled on the basis of relatively rough and ready allocation of state and nationwide aggregates and relationships.

The Berman input-output-based model of the economy of the New York metropolitan region has a great many more cells for data on the public sector than does the Leven formulation.[4] Paradox-

---

[4] Barbara R. Berman, Benjamin Chinitz, and Edgar M. Hoover, *Projection of a Metropolis* (Cambridge: Harvard University Press, 1960), pp. 21–22.

ically, in execution, the data problems were a great deal less severe in the former than in the latter study. This is because the Berman model focuses on the demand for goods, with productivity relationships mediating between output and employment; given the total absence of this kind of information at the local level, it was necessary to resort to the data on national interindustry relations. The financial information required was quite simple, in contrast, and could be developed, albeit painfully, from official sources without heroic estimates. On the other hand, the figures on behavioral relationships used in the projections for the government sector *were* heroic estimates, based on much thinner information than one would need, even with minimal standards for the results, which can only be described as anomalous: the employment projections, the end-product of the model, for local government proved to be highly volatile and not at all credible.

To be sure, many other estimates for other sectors made in the course of any regional economic study are equally shaky. But the point remains that however abbreviated the treatment of the government sector in regional accounts, there are substantial unmet data needs. The set of subsidiary accounts developed by Burkhead (see the appendices to his paper, above) would automatically provide a great many of the data needed and useful in both input-output and income and product analyses of regional economics, in addition to identifying government activity in some detail and providing information for public-policy decisions. Moreover, these accounts would also permit a much less crude treatment of government, particularly in regard to distinguishing between derived and autonomous activity, especially of state and federal governments.[5]

2. THE DATA REQUIREMENTS OF BURKHEAD'S SYSTEM

We now turn to the data requirements of Burkhead's system. The only data which current reporting systems are designed to produce in any form are those in Column 3 of the appendix tables—revenue and expenditure of local governments, whether in the region or in

[5] See, in this connection, Federal Reserve Bank of Chicago, *op. cit.*, pp. 3–4.

the rest of the world, so that what is dealt with is the levels of program account and service, not transactions account and the income-generating effects of local-government activity. The sources of the data are the Census Bureau compilations and reports, published and unpublished, of local-government agencies.

There are numerous deficiencies even here: lack of comprehensive coverage of all local governments in a region; lack of comparability in definitions and classifications; inaccessibility of the data to potential users; tardy reporting, missing years, and changes in classification over time; incomplete detail of the kind specified by Burkhead, especially in regard to functional classification and character of expenditure. Following from all this is the need for a massive investment of the user's resources to pull the various strands together.

However, despite these deficiencies, these kinds of data must be classed as available. Improved Census and, to a lesser extent, state-government reporting on local-government finance makes this material increasingly available. For individual areas, the possibility of reducing the detail required (e.g., agriculture need not be broken out in most urban regions) for meaningful analysis is considerable. In smaller areas or those with simple local-government structures, the investigator can reasonably expect to be able to dig out what he needs. None of these comments, of course, is meant to reduce the volume of the researchers' cry for improvement of this quite ordinary financial information.

Next up in the scale of increasing inadequacy of data resources is information on state-government direct expenditure and revenue collected within the region (Column 4 in Burkhead's tables). Here there is scattered material available, for some states, some programs, and some collections of local governments. For example, sales-tax collections by county and/or municipality are commonly available, but data on other taxes are less frequently at hand, although there is a fair amount of unpublished information potentially available. The situation is somewhat less favorable for direct expenditures, in part because the data are generated by a variety of operating agencies, many of which are organized on district or area lines and do not easily match with the regions likely to concern account builders. The Governments Division of the Bureau of the

Census is planning to provide some state-direct-expenditure data by county in the near future, which will help considerably, since the data then will be comparable on a national basis. Beyond this, it is not unreasonable to press state agencies to exploit the data they already generate and to develop more such data.

Information on federal expenditure within the region (Column 7) is still more fragmentary. Some data on payrolls and contracts are at hand and more can be provided, although the detail is limited. The problems of geographic disaggregation are a good deal more difficult, both operationally and in concept, than for state-government outlays. But surely the possibilities for improving the situation are considerable and not enormously costly, although the improvements need to be undertaken on a national and government-wide scale.

Burkhead has suggested some of the conceptual thickets one enters in attempting to ascertain the regional origin of federal revenues. On a collections basis, considering only the geographic point at which taxes are paid, data are now available only for Internal Revenue Districts, usually one to a state, with the exception of individual-income-tax data, available for larger metropolitan areas. At some (not insubstantial) cost, other taxes and more areas could be handled in a similar way, but the anomalies of the payment procedure will become much more aggravating as this is done (that is, payment at locations other than that at which the taxable event occurs, ignoring the fact that the economic chain leading to the taxable event has further geographic complications). Nonetheless, the existing work on individual-income-tax data by region and the data available with some effort on federal-employment-tax collections by county could sensibly be supplemented by regional data on excises collected at the retail level (including those on communications services).

The categories of data discussed so far have in common a very important characteristic: they are or can easily be automatically generated in the course of the normal operations of government agencies which are not primarily in the research and statistics business. Local-government financial reporting and county coding of federal and state expenditures are not beyond the ken of the administrator. And a general principle which applies to all statistical development is that the quality, quantity, and promptness of reporting are far superior when the information flows naturally from program operations.

Unfortunately, the other types of information needed in Burkhead's scheme are decidedly "unnatural" from the standpoint of program operations. This does not mean that we need abandon all hope, but rather that we must devise new ways to get at the material. Breaking down local-government financial items into region and rest-of-world categories (Columns 1 and 2) seemingly requires a direct assault on the operating agencies themselves, via surveys, interviews, and digging around in the files, for one-time studies, or via establishing new accounting and reporting schemes which have virtually no relevance to ordinary agency operations (and hence are hostilely received and produce poor-quality data), for continuing information.[6] I see no escape from this, unless one or a few large-scale investigations can develop some convincing sets of internal-external factors applicable to a wide variety of regional situations. In practice, of course, users may rely on *ad hoc* guesswork estimates, but this is not a very satisfying procedure.

A different approach is indicated for eliciting information on the regional distribution of state and federal financial items which represent events which affect the region but do not occur within it (Columns 5 and 8). The major element here is the allocation of benefits from programs which are statewide or nationwide in performance, notably defense and governmental overheads. One way out, of course, is to pinpoint every outlay on the basis of the area of its immediate impact—a state prison's outlays are allocated entirely to the region in which it is located regardless of its service area, for example. This way too is not very satisfying.[7] The methodological solution no doubt is to develop indexes to use as allocators

[6] Clearly, here too the smaller the region and the less complex its structure of local government, the easier all this will be.
[7] It should be noted that state and federal expenditures in a region may benefit other regions, and thus expenditures in the region on transactions account plus rest-of-world expenditures for the region's benefit do not add to expenditures on program account; Burkhead's tables would need an adjustment column for subtracting expenditures in the region for extraregional benefits, to get an unambiguous program-level total.

for such programs, much in the way that federal expenditures have been allocated among the states.[8] The value of the results of this approach depends upon the degree of refinement in selection of allocators (and considerable refinement can be costly) and one's confidence in the judgment of those who choose the allocators.

3. THE NEED FOR IMPROVED DATA

We are all aware, notably from experience with the national accounts but also from the limited recent experience with such regional-accounts items as county-income data, that new types of available data themselves generate analytical and policy uses undreamed of a few years earlier; in effect, investigators exercise unconscious or conscious prior censorship on the basis of data availability in defining the scope of their efforts. Therefore, filling in the boxes in Burkhead's system of accounts, even in part, can be expected to provide raw materials for the solution of all sorts of problems that seem far removed from our consideration, in this connection, right now. But on the other hand, no single system of accounts can be expected to contain within itself all the answers to specific analytical questions, and additional *ad hoc* efforts always will be needed. The point is that we need a far better intelligence base than we now have, to begin with.

Some of the specific points noted by Burkhead illustrate this. For example, systematic information on the sources of property-tax revenue in any geographic unit would involve a set of accounts subsidiary to his set of accounts, which are in turn subsidiary to regional economic-activity accounts. This kind of information in fact is available in limited form for some states and more can be developed by the piecing together of fragments in still other places, but unless it can be sold to property-tax administrators as data required for their own functioning, supplemental inquiries will be the most likely source of this kind of data for years to come.

Similarly, the development of data, in a comprehensive and usable

---

[8] See, for example, Selma Mushkin, "Federal Grants and Federal Expenditures," *National Tax Journal*, Sept. 1957, pp. 193–213.

form, on the characteristics of the stocks of public and quasi-public facilities as a basis for intelligent capital budgeting; the extension of the accounts to quasi-public agencies functioning in lieu of and alongside governmental bodies; and the distinction of government activities between autonomous and derived outlays in the nature of things are likely to require supplemental efforts, on occasion and in particular places. They are rather unlikely to be comprehended in a continuously maintained system of accounts applicable to areas of all sizes and types.

Of course, in practice today, these are the kinds of data produced only through expensive, *ad hoc,* one-time efforts. One such effort was the year-long one at the Regional Plan Association to develop a 25-year capital budget for the New York metropolitan region, a projection of the investment in public *and* quasi-public facilities likely to be required between 1960 and 1985 by a region developing as projected in the economic study directed by Raymond Vernon. This then is a projection of *derived* government (and quasi-public) investment, which also is tied closely to land requirements. The results are indicated in Table 1.

What were the difficult data inputs in this subsidiary account, and what are the prospects for closing the gaps? In order of increasing difficulty, the principal data problems, and the prognosis for improvement, are:

1. Incomplete base-year and recent historical data on local-government capital expenditure by type of facility (in reasonable detail). The 1957 Census of Governments provided the only firm platform, complete and comparable in its coverage, but even here the detail was not entirely adequate for this specialized purpose. State-government reports on local-government finance, individual financial reports of particular large local-governmental bodies (especially special districts and authorities), and fragmentary data on specific programs were partial supplements. As indicated earlier, one can reasonably expect, and demand, considerable improvement here.

2. Very sketchy data, to use as a platform, on the regional distribution of state and federal capital expenditure by type of facility.

Here, too, while there are some conceptual problems, the basic obstacles to data improvement are mechanical and the intelligent application of relatively small additional resources can close a good many of the gaps.

3. Even more limited data on capital expenditure of non-governmental organizations. Here there are no conceptual problems, but instead organizational obstacles of major consequence, for there is

TABLE 1. Projected Infrastructure Costs of the New York Metropolitan Region, 1960 to 1985

(in millions of dollars)

Type of facility	Total	To accommodate growth	For replacement and modernization [1]	Governmental	Private
Transportation	18,850	13,460	5,390	18,660	190
Highways	14,700	12,390	2,310	14,700	—
Commuter railroads and transit	3,030	250	2,780	2,930	100
Airports and port facilities	1,120	820	300	1,030	90
Education	13,090	7,790	5,300	10,030	3,060
Elementary and high schools	10,040	4,990	5,050	7,750	2,290
Colleges and universities	3,050	2,800	250	2,280	770
Water supply and sewerage	4,210	2,230	1,980	3,570	640
Health and welfare facilities	3,560	1,670	1,890	1,720	1,840
Parks and recreation	2,750	640	2,110	2,750	—
Other [2]	4,180	2,630	1,550	2,570	1,610
Region total	46,640	28,420	18,220	39,300	7,340

[1] Includes needs for corrections of egregious existing deficiencies (e.g., elimination of water pollution under court orders).

[2] Includes miscellaneous types of public buildings and equipment, and churches and miscellaneous non-public community facilities.

Source: Regional Plan Association, *Spread City—Projections of Development Trends and the Issues They Pose: The Tri-State New York Metropolitan Region, 1960–1985* (New York, Sept. 1962), p. 47.

no formal reporting of any kind to a central agency for many of these non-governmental organizations. In most cases, the first stage in data improvement—reporting of primary data to a central agency—would require a *de novo* effort on the part of the central governmental body (often at the state level) which regulates, licenses, or financially assists the class of non-governmental organization concerned, to compel systematic reporting. A second hurdle would be to ensure that these primary data are then organized in a form usable to outside researchers, as well as to the regulatory body, particularly in regard to geographic disaggregation.

4. The virtual absence of reliable coefficients linking urban growth to dollar magnitudes of public and quasi-public investment requirements. This is closely related to the lack of adequate base-year and prior-year data on capital expenditure, as noted in (1), (2), and (3), above. A really good time series on all forms of regional capital expenditure, whether local government, state government, or quasi-public, in sufficient functional and geographic detail would permit the investigator to link experience with capital expenditures to growth patterns and to standardize for differences in price level and equality. However, in all likelihood, the variety of environmental circumstances plus the instances of deviant behavior within a single region would limit severely the ability to generalize sufficiently to develop reliable coefficients. What is needed is similar time series for a whole array of regions, which would considerably raise the price tag of the required data inputs. But, even if all this were done regularly in systems of regional accounts in many different regions, converting the data into investment coefficients is likely to remain the province of the occasional specialized investigator.

5. The absence of an inventory of the existing stock of facilities, to permit estimates of replacement requirements (and existing excess capacity) during the projection period. Here, one would expect that the planning and budgeting requirements of ordinary operating agencies as well as the needs of official planning and budget agencies would result in a large amount of data on the age, condition, and capabilities of existing facilities. In fact, a fair amount

of such information does exist in a variety of agencies, in part thanks to urban-renewal projects and community-renewal programs. However, the available information [9] suffers from a number of disabilities in most cases: the planning horizons of the agencies are often ridiculously limited; the information is often in physical, not dollar, terms and is not in a shape which permits the generalization involved in reducing it to our society's financial common denominator; even when in dollar terms, differences in standards and definitions restrict comparability among programs; the completeness of the data differs enormously among programs and, more importantly, among units of government, so that the development of inventory data for any collection of units—say, for a Standard Metropolitan Statistical Area—is exceedingly difficult. We may call for improvements here, citing the obvious operating advantages to public agencies, but it seems doubtful that much will be done, in absence of some powerful financial bait and/or some strong policy-related pressures, both coupled with new (regional) organizational forms.

6. The lack of systematic standards of performance and measures of quality for public expenditure. This is a general problem, affecting a much wider range of considerations than is dealt with here, and the conceptual difficulties are stimulating work elsewhere.[10] I only note here that the problem has a bearing on most uses and structuring of data on the public sector, including the reflection of the public sector in regional accounts.

4. THE NEED FOR REGIONAL ORGANIZATIONS

What then is the action program indicated, to develop better data for the public-finance sub-account? A number of lines of attack

---

[9] This should be in quotes; frequently the operating agencies are not at all enamored of making these internal data public.

[10] This was a recurring theme at the Conference on Public Expenditure Decisions in the Urban Community, sponsored by the Committee on Urban Economics of Resources for the Future, Inc., May 14–15, 1962. See especially the paper by Werner Z. Hirsch, "Quality of Government Services," in Howard G. Schaller (ed.), *Public Expenditure Decisions in the Urban Community* (Washington: Resources for the Future, Inc., 1963).

have been suggested above. First, at the federal level, continued improvements in the scope and frequency of data developed under the program of the Governments Division of the Bureau of the Census can be expected. Beyond this, there is clear need for more regional disaggregation of federal-government revenue and expenditure. Second, state governments can greatly improve their reporting of the finances of their political subdivisions, and they, like the federal government, must make a start on disaggregating geographically state revenue and direct expenditure. Third, the quality of local-government financial reporting, which deserves grades ranging from "C" to "F" for 98 per cent of the universe (with a few sports in the "A" and "B" categories), from the standpoint of most potential users, can be improved enough to help account builders substantially. Fourth, both state and local governments generate substantial amounts of unexploited by-product data, in the course of their day-to-day operations, which can be tapped to fill in many of the cells in the accounts. Making these data accessible on a comparable and systematic basis has a high priority. Finally, there will be many kinds of hard-to-develop data with specialized uses which necessarily will be left to the specialized study to uncover.

This sounds like a rather piecemeal and incoherent approach. It is clear that the crying need, from the standpoint of the accounts for any given region, is for a systematic and integrated attack on the problem, to sell administrators on the importance of the statistical by-product and to reduce the quite unnecessary degree of noncomparability. But to accomplish this calls for some new organizational forms. As badly as we need a greater federal effort in the area of regional accounts, we cannot expect federal efforts to provide all the data needed, in the required detail and geographic breakdowns (at least not in the near future). As Harvey Perloff has suggested, there is a parallel need for organizations to deal with local and metropolitan information and analysis.[11]

Such organizations are being considered or developed in numerous places with differing functions and organizational arrange-

[11] In "A National System of Metropolitan Information and Analysis," *American Economic Review*, May 1962, pp. 356–64, esp. p. 364.

ments—Philadelphia, New York, Washington, Tulsa, to name just a few. It seems obvious that the mere warehouse of vast volumes of undigested miscellaneous regional data made feasible by the computer will contribute little either to the construction of regional accounts or to their application to analytical and policy problems. Rather, the need is for regional units, or groups of affiliated units, which will collect, tabulate, and store the scattered fragments in a coherent and retrievable form, will contribute substantially to the improvement of the quality, coverage, and comparability of data generated by others, will develop a system of periodic reporting of the general-purpose data developed and collected, and will utilize the information analytically.

It is likely that such regional data centers, information units, or what have you can make their largest contribution in the area of data on the government sector of the local economy. This fact reflects the relatively poor quality of existing regional data on the public sector (compared to existing regional data on employment, housing, population characteristics, financial institutions, etc.) combined with the fact that the supply of unexploited primary data which can be tapped at reasonably low cost is mainly that concerned with governmental revenue and expenditure programs. For many other data needs in regional accounts, considerable improvement over present conditions will require generation of new primary data, which is expensive.

It should be added that a regional unit, tailoring its activities to the specific research and policy needs of the region it serves, can also undertake the development of the types of data pessimistically assigned earlier in this paper to the *ad hoc* specialized investigation, if the region is intent on developing a comprehensive set of public-finance sub-accounts, without being hobbled by the fact that many of these data are not needed by regular operating agencies.[12] Thus, the conclusion is that the first order of business in data improvement for the government sector is not specification of a list of new series, but rather the development of well-conceived, curiosity-filled regional information and analysis organizations.

---

[12] For example, data on local-government expenditure within and outside the region, for the transactions, income-generation account.

COMMENT

LYLE C. FITCH
Institute of Public Administration

I have no comment on Netzer's excellent paper, as such, and will dwell upon the problems of getting some stuff for boxes whose emptiness we all deplore. Many of the basic data needed for construction of "economic accounts" for municipal and other governments are around; the problem is not one of starting to gather completely new data in an unexplored land. I do not mean by this that the problem of putting data into the required form is to be taken lightly; indeed, it might be argued that we would be better off if we were breaking new paths, instead of having to confront long-established accounting institutions manned by the more unimaginative members of a congenitally unimaginative race, that is, the accountants.

The accountants, by and large, have not been trained to think in terms of the requirements of economic analysis, planning, or developmental decision-making; their primary concern is an accounting for the receipt, disbursement, and custody of funds, down to the last one-hundredth of a dollar, and in recording the correlative asset and liability positions of their respective governments. "An accounting system of a governmental unit," says Tenner, "is designed to show not only financial position and operations but also the extent of compliance with legal provisions. The two most important legal provisions affecting governmental accounting are those relating to budgeting and funds." [1]

The accounting systems of local governments typically have little

---

[1] Irving Tenner, *Municipal and Governmental Accounting*, 3rd ed. (New York: Prentice-Hall, Inc., 1955), p. 3.

concern with the questions of fiscal policy, economic development, and other matters relating to over-all levels of activity and the government's share thereof. The deficiencies in governmental accounting, from the economist's viewpoint, stem not alone from the fact mentioned by Burkhead and others that there is usually no legal regional entity corresponding to the region for which accounts are desired. They stem also from the fact that, even in very large local governments like that of New York City, special information which the classification presented in Burkhead's paper would yield often is not desired, or, when desired, is manufactured in ways which leave plenty of room for argument over the details.

In the context of my own recent political experience, I have my moments of wondering whether information would be welcomed if it were "scientifically" compiled. To illustrate: One of the perennial arguments between New York City and New York state is over whether the city is in some way being "shortchanged" in the allocation of state grants to local governments. The contenders can seldom even agree on what the concept of "shortchanging" means, let alone on the amount thereof. One of the numerous expert attempts to go into the question was made about 10 years ago in a study of New York City finances for the Mayor's Committee on Management Survey;[2] the findings were abused by the city and more or less ignored by the state, which didn't want to set any dangerous precedents, and the argument went on as merrily as before. The point, of course, is that this is a question which can be greatly illuminated by a system of governmental accounts on the Burkhead model, but even if such accounts existed they would probably not be accepted in the way that measurements of national income are accepted, as utterances of the Delphic oracle.

Putting New York City's accounts into classifications which would facilitate preparation of an economic accounting statement for that city alone would be a substantial step forward in the New York City region, but one facing enormous institutional obstacles. And to follow through in the New York state sector of the New York

---

[2] Robert M. Haig and Carl S. Shoup, *The Financial Problem of the City of New York: General Summary Volume of the Finance Project*. Report to Mayor's Committee on Management Survey (New York, 1952).

region would probably require an amendment of the New York State Uniform Accounting Act, against the opposition of the budget directors and controllers and other municipal accounting functionaries, who would not be able to understand the implications of the new requirements and hence would oppose them; after which, if a New York attempt were successful, one would have to go to work on New Jersey and hope to get a similar framework adopted there, in an equally uncongenial environment. If the data coming up from the local-government units were properly classified, of course, they could be aggregated with little trouble. Many of the classification requirements are rather simple, once the system is installed, but there would always be problems, such as distinguishing between intersector and intrasector transfers, which would be formidable for the village bookkeeper. It is likely that some of the data forthcoming from smaller governmental units would not be of much value in any case. In this connection, most states now have some kind of uniform local-government accounting and budgeting requirements (which usually are not enforced), but the requirements as to form and procedures vary widely from state to state.

To make progress on regional accounts we must look first at data collection. We have two main alternatives, it seems to me, either to go after modifications in government accounting systems which will yield data in the desired form, useful for aggregation, or to persuade the Bureau of the Census, which really means persuading the budget directors and congressional appropriations committees, that this is a good thing to undertake. The first approach, I fear, is hopeless.

In the absence of any burning desire for data required by Netzer and Burkhead on the part of the people who have to gather it, and on the part of those who should be using it, what can be done? The Governments Division of the Census Bureau comes immediately to mind; in fact, the Census Bureau's own classification scheme is useful for some purposes but not for all, resting as it does largely on a cash inflow-outflow basis. The published Census reports have many deficiencies, of course, but the Census collects most of the basic data needed for a modern system of local-government-accounting reports. Another problem is limited coverage; annual reports are provided for three large cities of the New York metropolitan region—Newark, Jersey City, and New York—but owing to Census difficulties with terminology the village of Hempstead, L.I., larger than either Newark or Jersey City, is not shown in annual reports, and neither are the other 1,400-odd governments in the New York region.

To go back to the problem of modernizing specific accounting systems: there are required some changes in account structure and classification, and more work in data classification than most local-government accountants are accustomed to. I once was concerned with a project of this kind in Puerto Rico, as consultant-director of a project for revising the Puerto Rican accounting system. This revision had to do not with the basic integrity of the accounting system, of which there was little question, but rather with adapting it to the purpose of economic analysis and different types of decision-making. The task involved, among other things, designing a conceptual framework and fitting individual expenditure and receipt accounts into the framework. The old system of accounts, as is usual in such cases, provided much of the information needed, but it was necessary to rearrange and renumber some of the accounts and add a few new accounts. In some cases, definitions were rewritten to improve clarity.

Introduction of an economic-sector classification was another innovation. The old accounting system did not report the sources of receipts and the destination of payments, and did not completely isolate interfund transactions. Consequently, it was never possible to ascertain precisely the amount of the government's transactions with the outside world, nor the amounts of the transactions of the various governmental sectors with each other.

To provide this and other information on the flows of payments in the Puerto Rican economy, and between Puerto Rico and the rest of the world, an additional classification of expenditures and receipts was introduced. Receipts are classified and coded according to the economic sector of their origin and expenditures by the economic sector of their destination. In the Puerto Rican case, the economic sectors include three commonwealth-government sectors, municipalities, and individuals in Puerto Rico; partnerships, corporations, and sole proprietorships in Puerto Rico; individuals and business firms abroad; the federal government; and other foreign governments.

One economic sector was public corporations with independent treasuries, which kept their own accounts. There was considerable difficulty in getting them to assemble data, classified by economic categories, for the three-sector consolidation.

The first phase of the Puerto Rican venture, including the rewriting of the commonwealth accounting manual, required some two years, including some five months of my own time and a good share of the time of the young woman who was promoted to being head of the systems division in the accounting bureau of the treasury while on this job, and two or more assistants. So it was no simple task.

No other state or local government to my knowledge has undertaken a similar job. Many of our colleagues in the governmental-accounting profession have not even heard of social accounting, and most who have heard of it do not understand it. We are going to have a considerable selling job to do, and it is not going to be done very fast. The place to begin, it seems to me, is with the organizations representing professional and governmental groups—the Municipal Finance Officers Association, the Council of State Governments, and so on, and the National Committee on Governmental Accounting, sponsored by a number of these groups. As a beginning, some articles in professional journals and appearances at professional meetings are probably indicated, along with some lobbying at the staff level.

AN ACCOUNTS FRAMEWORK FOR METROPOLITAN MODELS

BRITTON HARRIS

University of Pennsylvania

In preparing, presenting, and discussing this paper, I have had consistent difficulty in relating the types of problems with which I am at present most deeply concerned to any clear and intellectually satisfying definition of the term "accounts." In the strictest sense, accounts might be defined for present purposes as a consistent body of data concerning stocks and transactions measured in money terms and constructed on a double-entry basis so as to be in principle susceptible to cross-checking. In this strict sense, I shall have very little to say about accounts. For purposes of the discussion, it seems convenient to loosen this definition and to assume that "accounts" is a term that may be applied to consistent bodies of data collected and maintained on a current basis, but not limited to quantities measurable in money or necessarily constructed on a double-entry basis. Even in this more general context, I have some reservations about the applicability of accounts to the problems of intrametropolitan models.

I originally limited myself, in preparing this paper, largely to the aspects of work at the Penn-Jersey Transportation Study which bear directly on the problems of data and accounts. As a result, it would appear that Mr. Niskanen and I have exchanged places and each discusses the other's topic. This phenomenon has proved not to be unusual at this conference. Since he and I are in wide agreement, I am happy that he has written such a paper and find it necessary to emphasize below only one major point of difference. In editing the paper for publication, I have found it desirable to preserve the original almost intact, adding only a short introductory portion. This limited divergence of the published paper from the presentation at the conference represents indirectly an acknowledgment of the stimulation and assistance I received through participating in it.

In the conference discussions, it frequently appeared that there was substantially more interest in types of models than in the more mundane problems of developing data to satisfy the needs of these models. In this context, I feel that one aspect of research into metropolitan and regional problems received inadequate explicit attention. In regard to metropolitan areas in particular, it has long appeared to me that very little is known about the real consequences of many policies. In pursuit of many important but frequently partial objectives, it is possible for policy-makers to initiate processes whose indirect effects are unforeseeable at the time. Yet these indirect effects may be at least as important in the general framework of policy as the immediate objectives being pursued. The broad object of both well-intentioned policy-making and urban regional research should be to draw out and consider the consequences of all policies upon the problem as a whole and upon related problems.

1. EXPERIENCE OF THE PENN-JERSEY TRANSPORTATION STUDY

The Penn-Jersey Transportation Study has embarked on an extended project designed to do exactly this type of testing of the extended and long-term implications of policies, particularly transportation policies. This project has involved us intimately both in the theory of the metropolitan area, and models which express that theory, and in the collection and organization of large amounts of data, some of which might be suitable for accounts use.

In grappling with this approach, we have encountered many novel problems. We have found, for example, that the interregional linear-programming locational models are not directly applicable to a metropolitan area in which space is intensively used. They must in some way be drastically modified to account for the importance of position rents and of the intense competition for the use of land and structures. We have also found that the analysis of metropolitan policy does not follow the simple and suggestive scheme of Tinbergen, quoted at the conference,[1] partly because there is great interdependence among the target variables and among the policy instruments or control variables, and partly because these classes of variables overlap widely.

The model on which we are working is rather disaggregated both with respect to areas and with respect to activities and population groups. It is predictive rather than normative, and insofar as possible we are attempting to make the actual structure of metropolitan interaction quite explicit. The model may gain some predictive power from the fact that it is temporally recursive and irreversible. Changes are conceived of as taking place in relatively small increments and responding to conditions as they exist during the time period under consideration. Later time periods must accept for good or ill the decisions made in earlier time periods. This approach and some further breakdown of the model, as for instance between residential and non-residential location, permits us to deal more readily with non-linearities, lags, and other complexities of the metropolitan area.

The over-all structure of the model and the way it may be applied for one particular time period and recycled for later time periods have been discussed in Penn-Jersey literature and circulated in the field.[2] A flow chart subsequently developed at RAND Corporation, and included in Mr. Niskanen's paper, parallels our own thinking remarkably and may be taken as giving a good overview of a model which we feel is appropriate to the metropolitan area.

The model which we are pursuing, unlike the RAND model, uses a linear-programming formulation, at least for residential location. This permits us to generate position rents directly. These position rents may be an important means of communicating between dis-

[1] See Karl A. Fox paper, above.
[2] See PJ Paper No. 4, *Topics in the Regional Growth Model: I*, by V. V. Almindinger.

crete parts of the model, and their changes over time are a most important means of evaluating the welfare indications of planning alternatives.

2. THE IMPORTANCE OF WELFARE ASPECTS OF PLANNING

It seems to me that in a technical discussion of accounts it is perhaps easy to lose sight of the importance of these welfare aspects of metropolitan planning. There is here a convergence of several considerations. First, when a metropolitan area is planned, residential accommodations and associated facilities are allotted well over half of the land area, and probably the nature, history, and development of these facilities and their utilization establish most of the real-world matrix for our present metropolitan problems. Second, while we tend to place emphasis on many public services and other non-monetary aspects of family welfare, it is quite clear that metropolitan planning can directly affect the pocketbooks and budgets of families mainly through the provision of transportation and housing and their associated costs. Awareness of the situation is indirectly reflected in many comments and remarks at this conference touching on living conditions, the journey to work, and the functioning of the metropolitan labor market. While this focus is thus by no means absent from the thinking of those at the conference, there are probably two pitfalls in considering metropolitan accounts and their utility which we should be careful to avoid. The first of these is a tendency to be interested in accounts which are most easily constructed out of data which is most readily available, regardless of its relevance. I agree with the remarks of Dr. Netzer that immediately visible relevance should not necessarily be a criterion for establishing accounts. The second pitfall may be a preoccupation with somewhat "flashy" public policies whose welfare implications are immediately apparent, or at least pretend to be so. This preoccupation could lead to a neglect of policies whose long-run implications may indeed be more powerful and more fruitful.

3. THE CONSTRUCTION OF REGIONAL ACCOUNTS

As a result of the foregoing concerns, I believe that I shall put forward the broadest set of demands on the construction of regional accounts. In some respects, the point of view which I represent is orthogonal to the interests and views of others concerned with accounts in the metropolitan region. The basis for these differences probably lies not in our views of research and of decision-making, but rather in the nature and scope of the problems which we are proposing to examine. I assume that I have been charged with relating the analysis of intrametropolitan locational tendencies to the accounts framework. It may well prove that this relation is so tenuous as to be inconsequential; but I shall begin by assuming that it is not so. This assumption will lead to the specification of a certain set of accounts. Whether such accounts are meaningful for other purposes, I leave to others to decide.

There would probably be wide agreement that the researcher into urban affairs and the policy-maker in the metropolitan environment are both concerned with the problem of making conditional predictions. Such predictions can, in general, be made only on the basis of a theory. A formal statement of a theory is identical, in my opinion, with a model. At the point of model-building, however, it is frequently necessary to abandon portions of a theory in the interests of feasibility. That is to say, a model may be an application of an incomplete theory, even when the model-builder "knows better." I specifically exclude from consideration any model which relies on the prediction of trends, since its assumptions must by definition preclude the possibility of conditional prediction under radically new policies or conditions.

Since field experiments designed to test theories of metropolitan development are egregiously expensive, and since the historical development of cities has not provided us with a very wide variety of controlled experiments, the necessity for experimenting on paper, both to construct theories and to make conditional predictions from them, is compelling. There is thus strong interest on the part of both scientists and policy-makers in the construction of models of metropolitan function. The construction and testing of theories and the making of predictions require data—for both inductive and deductive reasons. That is, available data about the metropolitan system, suitably organized, will suggest to the investigator hypotheses as to the nature of this system and the manner in which it functions. At a later point, when a theory has been formulated, data are needed to back up analyses designed to provide parameters, and to provide information as to the state of the system at the point in time from which conditional predictions are to be made. For a complex and elaborate functional system such as a large metropolitan area, and for certain types of theories, the data requirements may be very large and complex. Certain data requirements may conveniently be met by an established set of accounts.

I think that we may usefully distinguish several different levels of inquiry regarding the metropolitan region, to which different types of accounts and other data appear to be appropriate. The first and simplest level might be called "diagnostic." At this stage of inquiry, the approach is almost entirely inductive. The objective is to collect those indicators of metropolitan activity and welfare which will make it possible to provide a reasonably patterned and well-defined profile of the activities of a metropolitan region; of incomes which these generate; of the population, its composition, and its living conditions; and of the development of these indications over time. A second level of inquiry may be added to this one with an attempt at broad spatial distinctions within the metropolitan area. Insofar as these distinctions are limited by pre-existing data, they tend to contrast the central city with one or two "suburban" rings. A third level of inquiry might be called an aspatial interaction analysis. Carried to various degrees of sophistication, such an analysis would probe, for the metropolitan area as a whole, into those social and economic interactions which permit the area to discharge its functions internally and in the national and regional framework. A conventional metropolitan economic base study partakes of this character, as do to a very considerable extent studies such as have recently been carried out by Raymond Vernon for New York and Edgar M. Hoover for Pittsburgh. A fourth level of inquiry results from combining the second and third levels but still using rather broad areal units. Both the above-mentioned studies actually reach into this field, although the major emphasis of the Vernon study, at least, is largely aspatial within the New York metropolitan area. A fifth level of inquiry attempts to expand the areal detail of the second and fourth levels to the extent needed to arrive at relatively fine grain predictions with respect to metropolitan development patterns.

4. THE ROLE OF SOCIAL ACCOUNTS

We are now in a position to begin an examination of the role of social accounts, either scientifically oriented or policy-oriented, in the metropolitan scene. I think that three major but preliminary points deserve careful attention. First, accounts should not be relied upon to provide all information needed for any purpose, but should be restricted to purposes for which accounts are best suited. Second, the content of accounts must be appropriate to the level of inquiry in hand. Third, since accounts are conceptually constructed by the aggregation of "transactions," questions of detail which will arise in this discussion are not always as intractable as they may at first appear to be.

There are many questions, some of which loom very large in the analysis of intrametropolitan affairs, which are largely irrelevant to the construction of accounts. These questions are mainly behavioral in character, and answering them presupposes a theory of behavior in the relevant field. Thus, for example, the expenditure patterns of political jurisdictions might be described by a theory in political science, the locational preferences of households might be described by a theory in sociology, and the locational patterns of business concerns might be described by a theory in regional science or economic geography. These theories would be built upon microstudies of the behavior of decision units and would require a set of related accounts only to deny or confirm consequences which might flow deductively from them. An analogy exists in the case of national income accounts, which, no matter how detailed they may be, do not provide a basis for a dynamic theory of the response of producers, consumers, or investors. Such a response may be postulated for insertion into a model which makes use of or is tested by magnitudes compiled in accounts. But the origin of the postulate is observation and analysis of the behavior of economic units at the micro level, or speculation regarding it. These considerations lead me to emphasize the fact that in many cases the accounts information which might be made available for metropolitan models does not provide a basis for solving some of the major problems of constructing such models. For this purpose, much specialized supplementary information is required.

On the other hand, it should be clear that when specialized submodels which adequately explain some aspect of behavior have been constructed, accounts data can provide a useful basis on which they can be operated. For example, our knowledge of the behavior of individuals in utilizing an urban transportation system is rapidly becoming quite satisfactory as a result of a number of very expensive origin and destination studies. These studies have not yielded accounts data, but they have yielded a necessary theory applying to a part of the metropolitan system. This theory could in principle operate mainly on some of the more detailed accounts described below and reproduce with reasonable accuracy the results of an expensive O–D survey. In some circles, there is a strong feeling that transportation studies should move in this direction.

There is room for a major difference of opinion in the construction of metropolitan accounts which is based, it seems to me, largely on a difference of purposes. The spectrum of these purposes was sketched above. If it is desired, for example, to measure only governmental activity and its broad effectiveness for comparisons between metropolitan areas, a very limited span of accounts will suffice. Government fiscal data and some performance data are generally available annually and could be maintained in account form for any small set of areas at relatively little expense. Data on economic activity can similarly be secured at regular intervals, possibly annually. Data pertaining to population variables are more difficult to secure and are available in detail only decennially. It is relatively simple in most areas of the country to differentiate between broad rings within the metropolitan area on the basis of statistical data of these types.

The moment we attempt to extend the purpose for which accounts are constructed in any direction from this minimum, we encounter difficulties. If we attempt to measure in any serious way the interactions between sectors of the economy, we are handicapped by the lack of any flow data, a situation which prevails nationally as well. Within a local economy, we will find the lack of information as to flows between producers and consumers of the services of land and buildings to be a most grievous shortcoming. It seems likely that a number of special studies of the flows of goods and services in metropolitan areas will ultimately have to be made as the basis for the development of a theory which can provide adequate simulation of these flows, just as transportation studies now provide an adequate simulation of the flows of persons.

The accurate simulation of transportation flows involving persons and of interindustry flows or intersectoral flows involving goods and services gets us ever more deeply into spatial distributions. The very nature of interaction requires overcoming spatial separation. It seems very doubtful to me that accurate predictions can be made even on a broad basis of areal definition without a more finely structured analysis, and hence a more finely structured set of accounts, to build on. I consequently regard the fifth level of inquiry as appropriate and necessary, even for many purposes which are nominally covered by other levels of inquiry. Granting for purposes of discussion that we will consider accounts geared to this level of inquiry, let me make certain major observations about the composition of these accounts and the manner in which they may be established and maintained.

5. THE COMPOSITION OF ACCOUNTS

In contrast with most other social accounts, these will deal much more frequently with stocks than with flows. Even certain magnitudes which are in fact flows will tend to be regarded more as stocks for many purposes. Thus, business employment in various locations is from the social-accounts point of view basically an annual flow of labor services. From our point of view, however, it represents a stock of jobs in a particular area. Similarly, income may be appropriately regarded as a stock of purchasing power available in a given time period. Much more clearly in the realm of stocks in the strict accounting sense are the stock of housing, the stock of population, and the stock of productive facilities and capacity which are areally located within metropolitan areas. These locational stocks give rise to two types of flows, not all of which will in general be actually observed and made the subject of accounts. On the one hand, the daily interaction between the functions represented by these stocks leads to flows of people, goods, services, taxes, and so on. Most of these flows must be simulated. On the other hand, "migration" of components of these stocks takes place less frequently but permanently affects the distribution of the stocks. The status of these stocks, unlike that of economic stocks (except in bonded warehouses), is vitally affected by the mere passage of time, since a change in the age of a population represents a change in the population itself.

6. THE IMPORTANCE OF LOCATION

In discussing accounts in their simplest aspects, I have already begun to introduce the concept of location and to justify it. It is agreed that many of the most important policy questions which arise in metropolitan areas arise out of the differential distribution of activities (including residential location) and the interaction between these distributions. The structure of accounts which are designed as a framework for analysis related to these questions therefore must have a locational dimension. The problems of establishing the framework for this locational dimension, collecting data, and maintaining files are very substantial, and I relegate their detailed discussion to an appendix. Suffice it to say at this point that the locational aspect of accounts should have several desirable features. Locational aggregates or areas should be stable over time to permit intertemporal comparisons. Census tracts have not had this characteristic, but may acquire it. Areal units should be relatively small and of comparable size according to some such measure as geographic area, resident population, or total employment. This criterion disqualifies political jurisdictions because of the disproportion in size of the center cities and some other units. If possible, the areal units which specify location should be so defined that other existing data may be aggregated to these units. Because of the importance of population data and their inaccessibility below the census-tract or enumeration-district level, this last criterion suggests that area aggregates should in general be census tracts or groups of census tracts.

At this point, a distinction must be drawn between the locational designation given to observations and that given to aggregates. This distinction is important in gathering, processing, and updating primary information for which a more precise location is available than that provided by the system of aggregation. All too frequently, this additional information is discarded in the process of coding. It then frequently happens that at a later date, when a new system of aggregation is desired, the primary data cannot be reprocessed without very considerable expense.

The locational dimension is not the only dimension in which intrametropolitan accounts differ in general from the usually defined economic accounts. Economic accounts usually have a single metric, dollars, whereas social accounts have many dimensions, such as education, skill, race, status, age, sex (for populations); height, construction, dilapidation, and site coverage (for structures); and slope, elevation, drainage, and soil type (for land). One of the more important aspects of the metropolitan scene is that the dimensions of these different objects of observation are in various ways interrelated. Further, the variables pertaining to any one object of observation are interrelated and not independent. Thus, in fact, the dimensionality of these categories is less than the number of variables usually recorded. The structure of a set of accounts must take into consideration not only location but also a relevant set of dimensions for each category. Casting these dimensions in accounts form might lead to some quaint terminology.

Births and deaths become population flows, and education is a flow which increases the stock of status and earning capacity. Thus the formal structure of accounts of populations in the metropolitan setting suggests certain major divergences from the conceptual framework into which accounts were originally fitted.

7. FOUR KINDS OF ACCOUNTS WHICH SHOULD BE KEPT

There are four major populations or classes of objects of observations on which accounts should be kept in a metropolitan area. These are the land; the structures on it, including residences, business, and governmental structures; the activities which occupy these structures; and transportation facilities. This classification, however, does not accord well with the methods of collecting information, and for this purpose a slightly different format is desirable. This format would call for a census of resident population, a census of land and improvements, and a census of establishments, business, government, and institutional.

In many ways, the inventory of the resident population presents some serious difficulties. This inventory is taken only decennially, and intercensal changes are very difficult to estimate. The units of areal aggregation are arbitrarily defined (although not without reason) and are outside the control of the social accountant. The data, while presented in marvelous detail, nevertheless cover up some of the most interesting and important associations of variables at the level of the individual or the household. Such associations can be inferred only very unreliably from area aggregations, and their direct study is very difficult and costly. Despite these problems, I should not recommend any changes in the accounting for the location of population and its characteristics beyond what may be reasonably hoped for through the Bureau of the Census.

A locational inventory of activity and employment is difficult and troublesome. In the foreseeable future, however, state Bureau of Employment Security data can be locationally coded and tabulated as the basis for an inventory of economic activity by location.

The data suffer from deficiencies in coverage and inaccuracies of location for multi-plant employers, but in general these problems can be overcome. Since the location of employment can be inferred from the source information to the most minute desirable detail, there is in principle no reason why these data cannot be maintained in a form suitable for aggregation to any area breakdown. Once such inventory has been achieved for any given year and a system of file manipulation established, relatively limited additional work would be required to provide annual or biennial reports of the same type.

By far the most arduous new data-collection activity revolves around the establishment of an adequate land-use inventory, that is, an inventory of land and structures. Any agency entering upon precision work in this field has almost invariably found it necessary to conduct such an inventory afresh. Within a few years, it should be possible to establish standards and methods at such a level that one complete inventory of this type will be usable far into the future, and by the use of sampling techniques combined with administrative records of building permits and building-occupancy permits, it may be possible to maintain this inventory at a sound level of accuracy.

Accounting for the location, quality, and size of transportation facilities is relatively simple, although such accounts are not usually set up except in connection with large-scale transportation studies. Once established, such accounts change very slowly and are relatively easy to update. Data needed for them are relatively highly concentrated in a few agencies. Procedures which apply to this account also apply to a few other accounts covering public improvements or capital investments which otherwise belong in principle in the land and land-development category.

8. SIMILARITIES AMONG COMPONENTS OF ACCOUNTS

In brief, therefore, we conclude that the components of a complete set of the major accounts needed as a framework for metropolitan models display systematic similarities. Except in the case of the decennial Census of Population, these accounts have rarely been completely established in any metropolitan area to date. The establishment of any one account for any one year is feasible and may be required for various particular planning purposes, quite aside from the utility of the account or accounts for model-building purposes. In the larger metropolitan areas, the expense and effort involved in establishing such accounts *de novo* are very substantial. Although in principle the updating of such accounts through the use of administrative statistics and sampling techniques is both feasible and desirable, the practice has not become well established, even in cases where suitable initial inventories have been taken. Such a procedure is ultimately needed to produce annual accounts, but its special importance lies in the desirability for many purposes of having accounts available for the same year. Since it will frequently occur that not all inventories can be taken in the same year in one place, some method of updating the oldest inventories is important. It may be possible that administrative statistics can be used also to backdate accounts. This step is especially important to establish a framework for studies where the coincidence between Census material and other accounts is desirable but where it is unfeasible to wait for a new Census. Obviously, backdating and updating the Census is not feasible in major detail, nor is the provision of intercensal estimates in the same detail, without a system of permanent registration of the population, a system which seems unlikely to be applied in the United States.

If our metropolitan areas had developed smoothly and in large chunks so that areas of aggregation were homogeneous with respect to land and improvements, they would be duller places to live in but easier places to analyze. Insofar as areas are structurally inhomogeneous, the aggregation of area data may mask an association between subsectors of the population of households or of businesses and the population of structures. This masking is similar to the masking of relationships between variables within the resident population or the business population which results from aggregation of any type.

It is important to note that in the process of establishing and maintaining accounts on the location of employment and economic activity on the one hand, and on land and structure conditions on the other hand, the primary data collected originally contain or could contain sufficient information to permit the matching of these data by location precisely. Similar matching is not practical at the present time in relation to Census of Population data except by access in some controlled form to a sampling of the original unaggregated tallies. The matching of information from different accounts is extremely important from the analysis viewpoint, but of considerably less significance from the accounts viewpoint. It seems impractical to conduct most of this matching in the process of collecting the original data, especially because field interviewers are not apt to be skilled in the observation of more than one population. I bring this matter up in order to suggest that, to the extent that those who construct accounts are concerned with the management of primary data, they should be aware of the seriousness of any decision to suppress the precise locational characteristics of the data and thus to destroy the possibility of cross-analysis between populations which I have discussed.

9. SUMMARY

It is now appropriate to sum up the implications of the preceding discussion. The theoretical analysis of locational tendencies within the metropolitan area is complex. The development of this analysis to a point where sound conditional predictions can be made as a guide to policy is incomplete. It is already clear that such development will require a great deal of detailed research. In principle, such detailed research would be greatly assisted by the establishment of a set of locational accounts which was congruent with the aims of the research. It is clear, however, that many of these accounts would be of little utility for other purposes, and that their maintenance on a continuous basis is too time-consuming and costly for the purposes of locational analysis itself.

The locational behavior of decision-makers in the metropolitan area is conditioned by certain major variables which should be maintained in accounts form. These major variables are the residence of population, the location of activities, the land and structures, and the channels of movement. Each of these populations can be, with some effort, described in accounting terms. Such accounts are urgently required for many important planning procedures aside from the complete analysis of metropolitan location behavior. In each case, the primary data are collected in very substantial detail and with precise locational information. The problems of casting up the primary data in account form vary from population to population and depend on the methods used for data collection. Problems of classification and aggregation are not trivial.

On the other hand, the complete analysis of locational behavior involves in its major portion work based on data not conveniently cast in the accounts framework. The short-term manifestation of this behavior is the interaction of population elements by movement and communication, which has been studied in some detail, especially with respect to persons' movement in the metropolitan area, and can be simulated on the basis of the four major sets of accounts discussed above. Its long-term manifestation is the redistribution, migration, and change of these populations. The analysis of this requires many detailed sub-models and the coordination of these sub-models into a simulation of the metropolitan land market and its mode of seeking equilibrium. Such sub-models should ultimately permit us to simulate such behavior as the release of vacant land to builders, the deterioration of the housing stock, the movement out of areas by populations owing to changes in the environment or changes in their own status, and the process of aging and transformation of populations themselves. The overall simulation of the land market should permit us to simulate the processes of development and redevelopment, filtration in the housing market, and invasion and succession of different areas. None of these simulations can be made possible solely on the basis of accounts information. But once they are possible, the four major accounts outlined above will, just as in the case of movement simulation, permit the application of the theory of location to any metropolitan area.

From these considerations it follows, I believe, that accounts in their application to metropolitan location play two major roles. First, detailed and extensive accounts are most likely to be established and maintained initially in connection with a major analysis effort such as would be conducted by a metropolitan land-planning agency or a metropolitan transportation study. In this case, the needs of analysis tend to raise the level of quality and detail at which the accounts are initially established. Second, the existence of accounts in certain major sectors should facilitate the application of metropolitan locational models and will thus be a major aid to policy decisions. Such accounts are already being used piecemeal and in uncoordinated fashion by planning agencies and public officials in cities of all sizes. The establishment of a further level of consistency, completeness, and continuity in such accounts will further facilitate this decision-making, with or without the use of models. The expression in models of an adequate theory of metropolitan form and development will result in still further improving the basis of such decision-making. The consistent use of models, requiring a consistent pattern of accounts, turns out thus to be a characteristic of sound policy-making rather than a characteristic of locational models themselves.

APPENDIX ON THE OBSERVATION AND RECORDING OF LOCATION

It goes almost without saying that the locational aspects of an intrametropolitan model are of overriding importance. The resolution of the conflict between the necessity for interaction and the costs of overcoming space friction provides the key to the differentiation of functions and the distribution of activities of various types within the metropolitan area. The most important problem in setting up intrametropolitan accounts is therefore how to achieve proper consideration and management of the location variable. This need affects both conceptual problems and data management in powerful ways, but in ways which have not been fully explored. Three main aspects are here set out.

First, location is frequently considered as a means of classification and as a basis for aggregation. This is in fact a somewhat trivial aspect of location from a theoretical point of view, but one which has received such very wide application and attention that its status is now quite elevated. In this sense location corresponds, for example, with the concept of industry in the Standard Industrial Classification. The object of such a classification in dealing with economic data is to define a "neighborhood" within which the population achieves a certain degree of homogeneity. The actual basis of industrial classification is multi-dimensional, involving at least materials used, process, nature of product, and end-use of product. From time to time industries are freely transferred from one group to another as their characteristics or the form of the classification change. Areal units defined by location and size are not subject to such ready reclassification. Their dimensionality is more limited. Their parts must be contiguous. Such areal classifications as make use of location to define aggregations are useful for accounting purposes only in the range where the locational characteristics are truly invariant. Thus for problems of locational analysis where the scale of factors operating is small, large-area aggregations are useless. In the case of population characteristics which vary independently of location, if locational factors have not sorted the population into homogeneous groups, then any location aggregation may be inappropriate.

The second and more important aspect of location arises out of the fact that location specifies the possibility of interaction with other parts of the environment. In this case, location is a continuous two- or three-dimensional variable which may be defined in terms of Euclidean space. It is important to realize that the metric of interaction is most likely *not* to be identical with the metric of location. Much of the effort of model-building in transportation analysis and in locational analysis revolves around an appropriate transformation of the metric of Euclidean space into an interaction space. This transformation problem introduces many other vexing problems which are beyond the scope of this paper, since they have very little to do with accounts. It does suggest, however, the importance of establishing accounts dealing with those variables (such as transportation and communication facilities) which enter into the transformation process.

It may be mentioned parenthetically that the elementary two-dimensional nature of the location variable introduces its own difficulties into data processing, data management, and analysis. There is, for example, no "natural" order for census tracts within a metropolitan area and there is no simple way to present a comprehensible picture of the areal distribution of a variable, that is, of its locational variation, without recourse to maps. Simple difficulties of this nature often are not foreseen by the economist, sociologist, or statistician who is not accustomed to dealing with locational problems.

The third aspect of location is perhaps a special case of the second. In discussing the second aspect we said that the locational variable defined certain relations with the total environment. More particularly, we may say that the locational variable places a point in a neighborhood and thus facilitates the analysis of the impact of the immediate surroundings of that point upon activities conducted at it. Here the problem of scale is very important. At the scale of regional interaction it may be sufficient to say that a point is located in the New York SMSA or in the Boston SMSA. At the scale of over-all transportation-systems design it may be sufficient to say that a point is located in a particular census tract. At the scale of redevelopment decisions and commercial location it may be necessary to say that a point is located on a particular block front. Interpreting location as a specification of the immediate relevant environment provides one rationale for the area aggregation of data as discussed above, but it does not completely justify it.

Having in mind these three fundamental aspects of location, we may turn our attention to some of their implications for data management and for the construction of accounts.

The ideal format for the collection of data relevant to intra-metropolitan locational problems would involve provision to each observational unit of a précis set of locational co-ordinates. These co-ordinates would be a variable of the observation like all other variables. They would provide a basis for aggregation in any particular direction and under a variety of classification schemes. Such a proposal is mainly relevant to information which is collected on a universe basis, and it is not in any case completely practical.

The smallest practical unit of area that can be used as a basis for establishing location is the city block, and this unit is in many ways very attractive. It has the minor disadvantage in certain types of analysis of having usually four different faces or fronts, which may vary substantially in their characteristics. There are offsetting advantages in its systematic character, in its relation to street addresses, and in the fact that it has been widely used for the tabulation of Census data. The task of transformation of block information to a co-ordinate basis in Euclidean space is not trivial but it is manageable. Types of data to which a block-defined locational variable may readily be attached include land-use information and population. The list of types of data could be extended to include information on the establishments surveyed in the Census of Business and the Census of Manufactures and utility installations and changes therein, many types of city administrative information, state Bureau of Employment Security data, etc.

Aside from the questions of principle involved, there is a compelling practical reason for establishing all-new records of an accounting type on a block or co-ordinate basis. It is that past records on which an analysis of trends will depend vary widely in the basis established for area aggregation. This variation is apt to continue in the future over time and as between different sources of information. If the basic locational information which is to be compared with other observations is available in the finest of detail, adjustments can be made to bring it into congruence with other, uncontrolled systems of area classifications. Without this basis for adjustment the life of the analyst is one of overwhelming frustration.

In any discussion of the importance of systematic fine-scale work with area data, it is necessary to emphasize the difficulty and expense of engaging in it on a satisfactory basis. The preparation of adequate maps and the reduction of information to a system of area correspondence tables involve (for any medium-size metropolitan area) a number of years of painstaking work. The establishment of such a system as will be consistent, readily updated, readily manageable, and susceptible to easy coding and machine processing is not easy. The maintenance of this system on a working basis requires substantial staff time and the cooperation of many agencies. The extension of the system to additional data is likewise demanding.

COMMENT

IRA S. LOWRY
The RAND Corporation

I found Professor Harris' paper exceedingly stimulating and almost too tightly packed with ideas. It will repay careful reading by anyone interested in either of the two issues he discusses: the potential role of accounting systems in intrametropolitan models, and the problems associated with the locational identification of accounts data.

Those of us who work with detailed spatial-structure analyses can only salute and second his comments on the location-coding of data. There is an enormous body of urban statistics that cannot be used effectively in such analyses either because its location-coding system was irremediably specialized to some peculiar scheme or because location identification, present on the original field records, was suppressed in the early stages of processing.

I might add that the credit for breakthrough in this field properly goes to transportation analysts. A handful of metropolitan transportation studies, conducted by imaginative researchers, has shown us the possibilities of a very simple device: location identification by coordinate grid. This highly flexible system has the further advantage of being almost free of implicit theory. Area units used in other data-gathering efforts have almost always embodied a concept of urban structure which limited the usefulness of the data for other researchers. Even the design of the census-tract system was greatly influenced by the "natural area" concept of the Chicago school of human ecologists, and today's census tracts are a compromise between a territorial unit and a population unit. The "central city—metropolitan ring" dichotomy used by the Bureau of the Census for many of its otherwise interesting cross-tabulations also reflects a theory of metropolitan structure.

It seems to me that the time has come for some professional body —perhaps the Committee on Urban Economics—to prepare a manual for grid-location coding and begin to sell the method to the various data-gathering agencies.

With respect to the kind of accounts framework appropriate for the analysis of intrametropolitan locational tendencies, Professor Harris's paper reflects, perhaps too strongly, the perspective of his present commitments to a certain type of locational model. Within that context, his remarks are unexceptionable; but it may be useful to enlarge the frame of reference.

Professor Harris concludes that this accounts framework should "deal much more frequently with stocks than with flows." In fact, the accounts he specifically recommends are of the nature of periodic inventories of stocks—of resident population, of land and improvements, of employment in business and other establishments. While in some instances such inventories can best be maintained current by transaction records, he does not appear to be particularly interested in using these records as a means of determining the processes by which the inventories change. Much more emphasis is laid in his paper on the importance of cross-sectional inventory detail that will allow the analyst to associate specific characteristics with specific households, land parcels, and business establishments. This interest on Professor Harris' part is simply one expression of his conviction that patterns of metropolitan development can be predicted only by a microanalytic model which begins with preference systems for individual locators—households, firms, etc.—and works patiently through the low-level interaction processes. I will readily grant that this is one strategy for model-building, but I do not think it is the only one, or necessarily the best. Other approaches imply a greater interest in flow data than he exhibits.

There are three major types of flows that are relevant to the analysis of metropolitan spatial structure:

1. Diurnal traffic flows, which alter the distributions of people and vehicles throughout the metropolitan area in a more or less cyclic fashion. These flows are in themselves important in the context of transportation-policy decisions. They also implicitly define the spatial structure of the metropolis by relating origin and destination of movement. This spatial structure is the manifest outcome of the low-level interaction processes that Professor Harris wishes to simulate.

These daily traffic flows have been subjected to analysis by enough metropolitan transportation studies that it is now, as Professor Harris says, possible to simulate them, given the inventory characteristics of land use, residential population, and business activity. The traffic models use stock-flow parameters called "zonal interchange formulae" rather than microanalytic models.

2. Status changes of locationally fixed entities. This includes changes in the characteristics of land use and structures, changes in activity (e.g., employment or output) levels of business enterprises, and demographic or economic changes in the status of households. In accounting for changes of this sort, one has an automatic double-entry system, since movement from one status to another is always accountable in the double-entry sense.

3. Inventory changes that result from geographic mobility of socioeconomic entities. Here one has the option of an open or closed accounting system. If his interest is limited to maintaining current inventories, the origins and destinations of movers need not be recorded; all that is needed is a record of inflows and outflows pertaining to each locationally defined stock. However, if one is interested in the processes by which the stocks change, there is a good deal to be said for identifying both origin and destination of movers, and there is always the possibility that usable stock-flow parameters will emerge from these investigations.

With respect to the daily traffic flows, it is my sense that we are not through with origin and destination studies. The emphasis needs to be shifted now to the movement of goods rather than vehicles. I can't see much chance of progress in building locational models for business enterprise until we know a good deal more about these physical commodity flows, and the less tangible communication flows.

With respect to status changes, it seems to me that the use of stock-flow parameters can be extended considerably in model-building. Vital rates are just this kind of parameter, and there are, I think, analogues for physical structures as well—deterioration rates, conversion rates, etc., specific to age and structure type.

With respect to geographic mobility, I have two comments: First, recorded flow data can give us a good deal of insight into the pace of redistribution of population and economic activity. It is also clear that mobility varies with inventory characteristics. This suggests some stock-flow parameters that might well be useful. Second, I think we do need more flow data which record both origin and destination of such moves. It is obviously not practical to maintain a continuous record, but sample surveys would be very helpful as clues to the processes of change. The sample, in this case, is better constructed as an exhaustive enumeration of selected geographical areas than as a geographically exhaustive survey combined with a low sampling rate. This is because mobility analysis *begins* with an array of cells (e.g., the origins of all movers now residing in a particular area), and if *further* classification is to be done, a high sampling rate is necessary to fill the cells of each added dimension.

THE USE OF
INTRAMETROPOLITAN DATA

WILLIAM A. NISKANEN
U.S. Department of Defense

Urban problems evoke various characteristic responses. Reformers call for more imagination. Politicians want more authority. Subdividers demand more land. Builders order more concrete and steel. And social scientists, with outward composure and some new-fangled techniques, ask for more data. This paper outlines a program for the organization and use of intrametropolitan data that may contribute to the solution of some of these problems.

Two developments during the last year illustrate the nature of our requests for more data on the regional and urban communities. Three prominent economists proposed major national programs to collect and analyze data on our subnational economies. Guy Orcutt proposed the development of a large microanalytic model of the United States economy, requiring the collection and analysis of data for each major region and structural component.[1] Harvey Perloff proposed a general framework for a national system of urban accounts.[2] Werner Hirsch proposed a more explicit framework for the analysis of the relations among regions and a comprehensive record of persons and property within each region.[3] The tenor of these proposals suggests that the problems have

[1] In "Microanalytic Models of the United States Economy: Need and Development," *American Economic Review*, 52 (May 1962), 229–40.
[2] In "A National System of Metropolitan Information and Analysis," *American Economic Review*, 52 (May 1962), 356–64.
[3] In "Design and Use of Regional Accounts," *American Economic Review*, 52 (May 1962), 365–73.

been identified, the techniques are developed, and the computers are ready to roll when the data are available. A second development contrasts sharply with these comprehensive proposals. Several communities are preparing to establish the first regional or metropolitan data centers. Initial funds were provided, largely by the Housing and Home Finance Agency, for a demonstration project in five Midwest metropolitan areas. These initial efforts have experienced two common problems—substantial disagreement concerning the objectives and activities of the data centers and an ambivalent response by local public and business interests. One questions whether a comprehensive national system of urban accounts should be designed until the experience of a few operating data centers is evaluated. One wonders whether these experiments will be valuable without more realistic guidance from the community of social scientists. With such guidance, local experiments with various concepts of the urban-data center may lead to a more general consensus concerning the urban communities' incremental demand for data.

Part 1 of this paper considers the value of an organized system of urban data for various public and private decisions. Part 2 outlines a model of the urban space economy and suggests the use of the model as a framework for organizing data and as a management tool. Part 3 discusses the organization of data within each metropolitan area and suggests a set of studies on behavioral relations that are common among areas. A number of criteria are implicit in the design of this approach:

(a) decisions to which the data contribute should be explicitly identified;
(b) maximum use should be made of characteristics which are common among urban areas; and
(c) the model should permit the use of a variety of analytical techniques, depending on the nature of the problem and the precision of the data.

These criteria are particularly important for the next few years, as funds for data and analysis in most urban areas are stringently limited, and regional science is still a mixed bag of tricks.

1. THE VALUE OF AN ORGANIZED SYSTEM OF INTRAMETROPOLITAN DATA

The value of additional data on our urban communities is equal to the increased cost of public and private actions taken in the absence of such data. The value of possible savings in other resources, if the additional data critically influence the decision and the full savings are realized, is clearly high. Most of us are guilty of writing research proposals which include a comparison of the millions of dollars which could be saved (pick your problem) and the modest cost of the proposed research. Our financial sponsors, however, reflect their subjective estimates of the expected savings in other resources by grants of a fraction of our requests. As long as there is a "shadow price" on funds for additional data and analysis, the allocation of research funds should be based on the relative marginal products of the various projects. We dream of riches and general equilibrium; we work with modest resources and partial equilibrium.

What is the case for a major increase in the data on our urban communities? A favorite introductory paragraph to current articles in this field describes the rapid growth of urban areas, but the demands for data have increased more than proportionately. In part, this increase is attributable to the reduced cost of data collection and processing—the result of more general understanding and use of sampling techniques and the use of electronic data-processing equipment. An organized system of urban data would contribute to both private and public decisions of major importance, but most of the recent demands for data, interestingly, have originated in the public sector. Three historical changes in the character of local government have contributed to these demands:

(a) a continuing trend from the general regulation of private activity (through the framework of civil law) to specific restrictions on private action;

(b) an increasing concern for the "indirect" effects of public actions on the characteristics of urban form;

(c) a larger scale of public services, accompanied by the belief that "big" decisions must be evaluated by different criteria and new analytical techniques.

Lowdon Wingo expresses a general evaluation of these changes, stating,

Perhaps the most significant aspect of this development is the change in intellectual demands posed by the new policy issues: increasingly they are issues which are not easily amenable to conventional design solutions but require new kinds of knowledge, new frameworks of analysis, and new criteria for making decisions. . . . The old trinity of "objectives, status quo, and plan" will not suffice to provide rational policies in an urban universe of interrelated private and public purposes and of intricately related developmental processes which can be irreparably disturbed by the effects of poorly calculated "big" decisions.[4]

Whether or not one is happy about these developments or agrees with this evaluation, both are part of the environment for the increased data demands.

Three general types of policy questions are generating the demands for additional intrametropolitan data and new analytical techniques:

1. How to evaluate the indirect effects of public actions, such as
   (a) the impact of a change in the transportation system on other elements of the system and on land use;
   (b) the locations of businesses and residences displaced by a redevelopment program or freeway construction;
   (c) the retail sales and land values in areas not directly affected by new public services.

2. How to project the long-run demand for public services from the spatial distribution of economic activity by business and household characteristics.

3. How to project the long-run tax resources available from the spatial distribution of retail sales, user charges, and property values.

[4] Lowdon Wingo, Jr., *Transportation and Urban Land* (Washington: Resources for the Future, Inc., 1961), pp. 2, 3.

Better impact evaluation and long-range projections would most benefit decisions on projects with a large fixed (economic or political) cost but would also contribute to the routine processes of program and budget planning.

2. A MODEL OF THE URBAN SPACE ECONOMY

A model of the urban space economy must necessarily focus on the distinguishing characteristic of urban form—the spatial relations among complementary activities within the urban area. A city forms and changes to realize both internal and external economies of scale; the resulting proximity of land use, however, is the basis for the unique urban problems arising from the divergence of social and private welfare.

A model based on these internal spatial relations could make two valuable contributions to an understanding of these problems:

1. As a data-organizing system:
   (a) The explicit identification of input, functional relations, and output suggests the gross data requirements.
   (b) The model formulation suggests the grouping of data by homogeneous behavior patterns.
   (c) Sensitivity tests may be used to identify the critical data.
2. As a management tool:
   (a) A model may be used to substitute for real experiments to test the impact of public policy. A model may sometimes provide more powerful tests than a real experiment because of the problems, in the latter case, of identifying the response to a specific action. A model will also be less expensive in dollars, votes, and time. One valuable by-product of a model formulation is often the suggestion of small-scale real experiments to buy information on public response.
   (b) A model may be used to forecast private actions as a guide for public decisions. The forecast period will depend, in large part, on the level of detail, but most estimates for periods longer than five or ten years, I suggest, have little meaning or relevance.

(c) A model may also be used as a sales tool. It is important to remember, however, that models, like advertising, can be used either to aid or to confuse popular understanding of a public program.

A city is a functional organism only in an evolutionary sense. At any point of time, its spatial structure is the product of past decisions, "accidents," and the conscious and unconscious maximization decisions of countless independent units. Over time, cities evolve toward a functional form, but "given conditions" are so massive compared to the changes occurring during interesting time periods that most cities only vaguely approximate an "optimum" or stable urban form. The simulation model outlined in this section reflects this concept of urban form; the structure of the model is based on the conjecture that the behavior of decision units making a change during a given time period is more homogeneous among urban areas than behavior of all such units. Cities change in much the same way, I suggest, when subject to similar conditions, but the over-all spatial form of a city is most strongly determined by past conditions.

The simulation model consists of four major components—status variables, input variables, functional relations, and output variables.

1. Status variables describe the spatial distribution of activity within the urban area at the beginning of a period and the constraints on decisions made during the period. There are eight general types:

(a) households,
(b) employment,
(c) physical structure,
(d) vacant land,
(e) transportation system,
(f) land-use constraints,
(g) position rents (optional),
(h) retail sales (optional).

2. Input variables describe the conditions originating outside the urban area and within the public sector during the period. There are four general types:

(a) new households with no wage earner,
(b) new employment outside of sales and services to internal business and households,
(c) changes in production and transportation technology,
(d) "exogenous" changes in public policy affecting land use and the transportation system.

3. Functional relations describe the changes occurring during the period from the input variables' acting on the status variables. There are four basic sets of functional relations:

(a) locator pools generate the total net movers within the urban area and the new locators, grouped by location behavior;
(b) location models distribute the net movers and new locators, grouped by homogeneous location behavior, among the subareas;
(c) transportation models generate and allocate the trips arising from the new distribution of employment and households among subareas, modes, and routes;
(d) status-variable modification routines generate the induced changes in the status variables arising from the new distribution of employment and households.

4. Output variables describe the spatial distribution of activity at the end of the period and, in turn, become the status variables at the beginning of the next period.

The general relations among these four components are illustrated by the chart (Figure 1). The structure of the model is similar to that of an economic base model, decomposed by homogeneous location behavior and subareas. Changes in total employment are derived from changes in "basic" employment, and changes in population are derived from the changes in employment. Functional relations within the locator pools and the business and household location models are direct independent transformations; the distribution of employment by industry and area, as a result, does not include any "induced" input-output or location effects within a given period. The employment-household-transportation sequence reflects the relative speed of adjustment to new conditions, but this sequence is quite arbitrary for "short" periods.

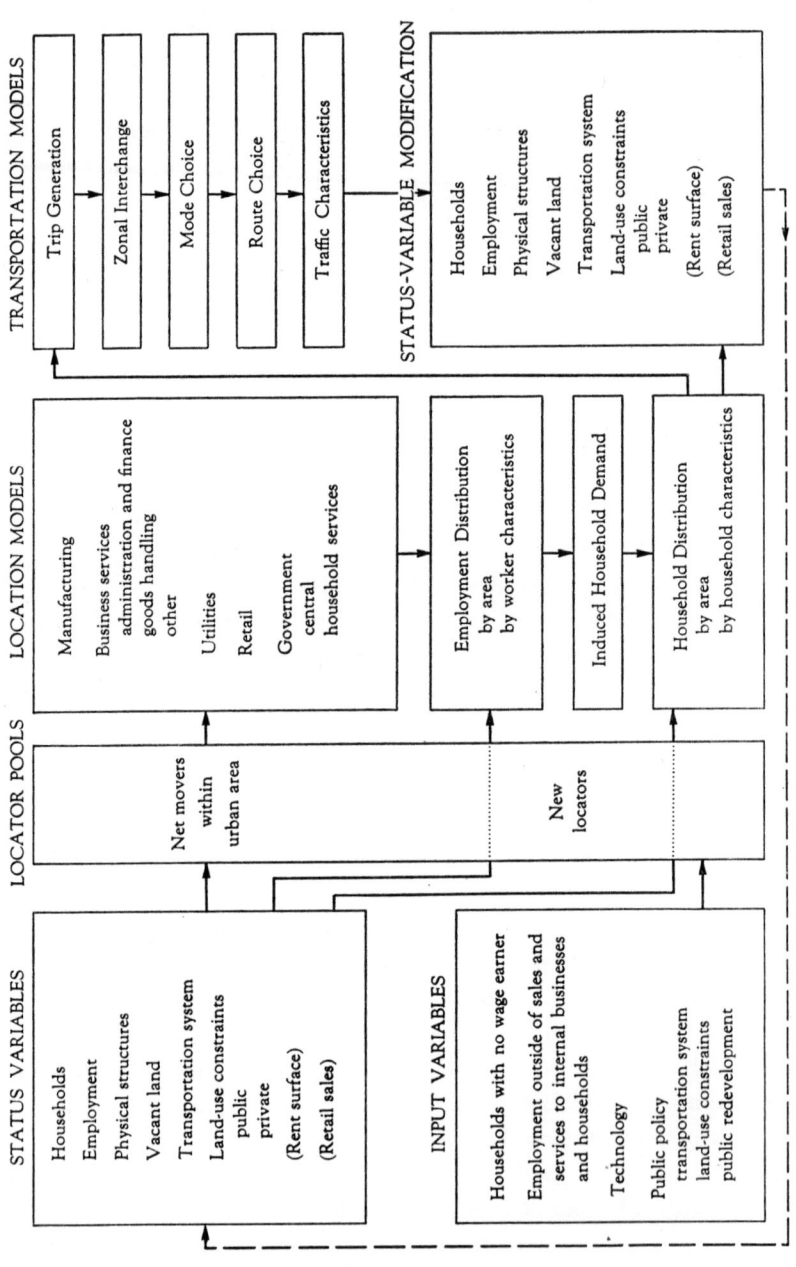

Figure 1. A Conceptual Model of the Urban Space Economy

Given this general structure of the model, there are three critical problems of model formulation: choice of the basic areal unit, choice of the iteration period, and choice among the major types of functional relations.

1. Choice of the basic areal unit will depend on the availability of data, limitations on the computer used, and the precision of the analytical routines. For a variety of reasons, I suggest that the basic unit for such models should be the lowest aggregation of census tracts which forms a meaningful submetropolitan community. The census communities, where such are identified, are appropriate, and political units can often be used outside the central city. For most urban areas, the number of such units would be from 50 to 200, so that sufficient areal detail would be provided for almost any metropolis-wide policy problem. Our analytical routines aren't worth a damn, in any case, for forecasting location on traffic conditions within smaller areas.

2. A short iteration period (say, one year or less) is most consistent with the recursive structure of the model outline. The model-builder faces the problem of accounting for the lagged effects over successive short periods or the effects of mutual determination within a longer period. Given the present status of our analytical techniques and the computer limitations, the lag problem is much less severe.

3. The most difficult problem of model formulation is the choice of functional relations. Two major types are distinguished: "structural" relations based on an explicit maximization model, and the "reduced form" relations derived from this model. The choice among these formulations depends on one's interest in the structural relations, whether information independent of the model structure is available on some variables, and the types of data available. Despite our professional interest in the structural relations suggested by a formal theory, they are often difficult or impossible to estimate, and the reduced-form relations usually provide better forecasts. A number of good model-builders have stumbled over the problem of incorporating position rents into a location model, but unless one is directly interested in these rents

(to estimate property-tax revenues or the impact of rent control) a fully satisfactory location model need not include this variable. The potential model, for example, has little interesting theoretical content but is probably the most powerful construct of regional science. There appears to be no need for a single analytical routine to solve all the functional relations. A variety of routines may be used, depending on the nature of the data available and the problem addressed.

A model of this nature cannot answer many of the questions of urban policy. It cannot forecast the input variables. It cannot provide the spatial detail that is necessary for precise land-use and transportation planning. It cannot substitute for careful cost-benefit analyses of public programs. The process of model formulation, however, clarifies one's outlook on these problems, and development of the model would provide a breakthrough in our understanding of the relations among submetropolitan communities.

3. ORGANIZATION OF THE DATA AND FUNCTIONAL RELATIONS

A rational organization of urban data will require a much greater specialization of interests and activities among regional scientists. Analysts of a particular urban area should be primarily concerned with the data and functional relations specific to that area. The broad group of regional scientists should be primarily concerned with the data and functional relations that are common among urban areas. At the present time these functions are disturbingly confused; each major regional study has had to develop a new set of functional relations, and the majority of regional scientists have not had the money or motivation to work on these building-block relations. Britt Harris' comments on the Pittsburgh study are widely applicable:

One might argue on principle against the necessity for a study like the Pittsburgh Regional Economic Study to review national location patterns, factor costs, and goods movements—on the grounds that such effort is duplicated from one study to the next. This is indeed true, but if the general framework of regional accounts does not provide this information such duplication will be forced upon various successive studies.[5]

The role of a local study group in developing a model as outlined above would be to collect the status-variable information, prepare alternative forecasts of the input variables, and update and revise the common functional relations to reflect the unique conditions of the area.

A local data center, possibly the type of information center envisioned by Ed Hearle,[6] would be responsible for collecting and organizing the following status-variable information by census community or comparable unit:

(a) number of households by age composition, sex of head, race, labor-force participation, occupation, and income;
(b) number of employees by industry and occupation;
(c) number of physical structures by size, type, and quality;
(d) amount of vacant land by size and potential use;
(e) capacity and time characteristics of transportation links with adjacent areas;
(f) nature and extent of the public and private land-use constraints—these may be grouped under (c) and (d) above;
(g) average position rents;
(h) total retail sales by major product and service group.

Each area would be described by about 100 of these attributes, so considerable detail in the important variables is feasible. The records of these status variables would not be "accounts," in the formal sense, since they would not be sufficiently complete for a consistency check or sufficiently frequent for impact evaluation.

A special local study group would generate alternate forecasts of the following input variables:

[5] Britton Harris, Comment on "The Role of Accounts in the Economic Study of the Pittsburgh Metropolitan Region," in *Design of Regional Accounts*, Werner Hochwald, ed. (Baltimore: The Johns Hopkins Press, 1961), pp. 271–72.
[6] Edward F. R. Hearle and Raymond J. Mason, "Data Processing for Cities," P-2492 (Santa Monica: The RAND Corporation, 1962).

(a) number of new households with no wage earner, by above household characteristics;

(b) new employment outside sales and services to internal businesses and households by industry and occupation;

(c) changes in production and transportation technology which would affect local conditions;

(d) changes in public policy affecting the transportation system, land-use constraints, property taxes, or public land uses.

As part of (b) above the local study group would also revise the common input-output relations to reflect the local conditions.

Development of a model such as outlined in this paper will depend most critically on the identification of functional relations that are common among metropolitan areas. Studies of the following types of functional relations are required:

(a) mover frequencies by function,

(b) location behavior by function,

(c) land use by function,

(d) transformation from occupational to household characteristics,

(e) trip generation and travel behavior by function,

(f) conditions determining the construction and maintenance of physical structures by function,

(g) conditions determining the release of vacant land,

(h) conditions determining the "induced" changes in public policies affecting transportation and land use,

(i) conditions determining the rent surface,

(j) the relation of retail sales to the distribution of purchasing power.

The major regional studies of the last few years have already made a substantial contribution to an understanding of these relations. Some of the required studies are under way at RAND, the Transportation Center, and elsewhere. Further studies of these relations, however, should not be deferred until a formal system of urban accounts is available. These studies will require data not provided by such accounts, and these studies, I suggest, will prove to be more valuable.

COMMENT

LOWDON WINGO, JR.
Resources for the Future, Inc.

Niskanen has set forth a model of the urban space economy as the appropriate vehicle by which intrametropolitan data can serve the metropolitan decision-maker. His discussion is clear and persuasive. If it fails to convince, it is because of an understandable tendency to cast the problem in the limited terms of a particular model-building experience. Pity the poor decision-maker who, stimulated by the possibilities which Niskanen has opened up, finds himself left with an untidy heap of interesting constructs, each of which, we aver, should help him to make better decisions and so to meet his responsibilities more effectively. Models, data centers, regional accounts, policy analysis, indeed, even rational decisions, will be increasingly urged upon him; a useful service, perhaps, is to be performed by urging upon Niskanen an extended framework more in keeping with the pace of developments in metropolitan policy-making.

Decision-making on the urban scene was not always so complicated as it will appear to the readers of these essays. Within our lifetimes several developments have sapped our simple-minded notions of cause and effect (and, consequently, of "problem" and "solution") in that elaborate behavioral system, the modern metropolis. Awareness of the complexity of urban phenomena has expanded rapidly while social, economic, and political relationships were becoming more intricate; at the same time, our involvement with processes of planning and broad urban policies has compelled the inclusion in policy calculations of an ever-increasing array of the consequences of alternative policies—has pressed policy-makers continuously toward higher-level suboptimization.

Almost no socially significant decision taken by public or private institutions on the urban scene is such a simple process as coping with a traffic bottleneck, for instance; that is, getting the facts and judiciously choosing a straightforward solution. More typically policy-making is a matter of mastering complex relationships, of understanding the consequences of alternative courses of action in terms not only of the characteristics associated with a particular problem but also of the policy side-effects which generate new problems. In the good old days we tackled the slum in a straightforward way by tearing it down. Now we know the slum to be a complex social mechanism of supportive institutions, of housing submarkets, of human resources intertwined with the processes of the metropolitan community as a whole. The nature of the urban housing market—and our incapacity to eliminate the slum-dweller with the same dispatch with which we can demolish the slum dwelling—insures that a strategy of demolition will intensify occupancy of remaining slums, put irresistible pressures on the old marginal areas, and levy against the welfare of the most defenseless and needful segments of the city's population. On balance, it would be difficult to demonstrate a net social gain, and all because the relationships among parts of the system or urban housing markets were ignored or misunderstood.

We are now prisoners of our discovery that in the city everything affects everything else. Notwithstanding advances in welfare economics and benefit-cost analysis, even to distinguish favorable policy outcomes from unfavorable ones is no longer a simple matter. Decisions by governments, firms, and individuals in metropolitan areas turn on the state of such interdependent spatial systems as use of recreation facilities, transportation and communication nets, and the markets for land, housing, and even labor, rather than on the highly localized consequences directly elicited by policy actions. The rapid evolution of a genus of mathematical techniques, or models, to conditionally predict certain locational aspects of the behavior of urban populations has been both cause and consequence of these developments. Metropolitan highway-planners simulate regionwide traffic flows in computerized networks through which they can follow the anticipated consequences to local changes in traffic facilities. The Penn-Jersey Transportation Study, the Pittsburgh Economic Study, the RAND Corporation, and others have worked toward models to predict the intrametropolitan arrangement of economic activities. Pittsburgh and San Francisco are pioneering the use of such models in urban-renewal policy-making. The metropolitan open-spaces study in Washington will use an econometric model to relate the spatial distribution of demands for recreation activities to the regional distribution of recreation areas and facilities. These are all intrametropolitan models concerned with various spatially interdependent aspects of regional growth and change.

What is suggested is that we should be talking not about The Intrametropolitan Model but about intrametropolitan models. Although Niskanen sets out for his approach the condition that the "decisions to which the data contribute should be explicitly identified," he later seems to be concerned only with a multipurpose, archetypal model. However, the specific needs for conditional predictions to inform quite particular kinds of regional policies are likely to encourage in the near future the construction of models of the urban space economy both *ad hoc* and partial. The immediacy of these tools for the policy-maker concerned with urgent decisions probably makes them of more interest to him at this moment than the more general models of the urban space economy.

Such models are likely to revolutionize the character of the policy analyses backing up metropolitan decision-making processes. Because intrametropolitan models focus attention on the city as a set of spatially interdependent behavioral systems, they will by indirection point out critical interdependencies among public policies. Already it is clear that the intrametropolitan structure of land use and that of transportation are tightly coupled policy areas. In the future the relation between slums and social-overhead investment, or between youth services and housing markets, or between recreation and transportation will become equally clear. In any case, policy formation will depend on increasingly specialized kinds of intrametropolitan analysis. Specialized information inputs will be demanded for the development of anticipated values for the output variables needed to inform decisions in these areas. Sophistication of policy analyses is virtually an inevitable consequence of the computerization of government functions, the introduction of the behavioral findings of the social scientist, the expansion of government functions in the metropolitan region, and the sheer growth in scale of metropolitan society. This is a force again carrying us in the direction of more specialized models of the metropolitan space economy.

How rapidly these developments mature depends heavily on the accessibility, rather than the availability, of a large array of data. Werner Hirsch has pointed out the *availability* of 90 data items on parcels, 103 on persons, and 35 on street and road sections in most Standard Metropolitan Statistical Areas. Extensive automation of local-government record-keeping and information processes supplemented by the development of metropolitan data and statistical centers promises to open up this immense vein of hitherto-inaccessible information for analysis of the critical functional relationships reflected in it, and for a running picture of the state of important intrametropolitan systems. Further, Albert Mindlin has proposed a continuing sample survey to provide current information on the state of such important regional stocks as housing and employment by small areas. A significant mission for regional accounting is implicit in this proliferation of information about persons, places, and the activities which link them—to provide the framework to organize the data in an information system. The successful carrying out of this responsibility can bring into play the more powerful analytical techniques to support the difficult and costly decisions confronting metropolitan decision-makers.

In summary, my quarrel with Niskanen's paper, if I have one, grows out of its reluctance to examine "the use of metropolitan data" in the broader perspectives which the rapidly changing context of metropolitan decision-making would seem to demand. The danger in the paper's perspective is that it could lead to commitments about the content and scope of intrametropolitan data that are too restricted, too simple, and too static for this rapidly changing context. It is, notwithstanding, a lucid, economical exposition of the information issues being encountered in the development of intrametropolitan models.

THE MEASUREMENT OF HUMAN RESOURCES IN A REGIONAL ACCOUNTING FRAMEWORK

LEO F. SCHNORE

University of Wisconsin

Traditionally the economist's interests were focused on the classical factors of production—land, labor, and capital. Today, however, we are confronted with an economic vocabulary that intermixes these older concepts, so that one finds frequent references to "human capital" and "human resources." [1] Whether or not these verbal innovations have any special merit in themselves, they do serve to point up a fundamental fact: *the quantity and quality of human population are coming to be vital considerations in most areas of economic analysis.*

More than changes in vocabulary and usage seems to be involved, for whole new specialties are being developed, with subareas devoted to particular population characteristics. Both "educational economics" and "health economics" appeared alongside "welfare economics" even before the creation of a federal Department of Health, Education, and Welfare.[2]

---

[1] Theodore W. Schultz, "Investment in Human Capital," *American Economic Review*, 51 (March 1961), 1–17; and his "Investment in Man: An Economist's View," *Social Service Review*, 33 (June 1959), 109–17; see also Eli Ginsberg, *Human Resources: The Wealth of a Nation* (New York: Simon and Schuster, 1958) and Dael Wolfle, *America's Resources of Specialized Talent* (New York: Harper & Brothers, 1954).

[2] Selma J. Mushkin, "Toward a Definition of Health Economics," *Public Health Reports*, 73 (Sept. 1958), 785–93; Rashi Fein, *Economics of Mental Illness* (New York: Basic Books, 1958) and Alice M. Rivlin, "Research in the Economics of Higher Education: Progress and Problems," processed manuscript, 1961, 53 pp.

One may venture some guesses concerning the reasons for these developments, which seem to represent more than mere academic fads. Ultimately, they appear to stem from the recognition of certain salient social problems confronted by advanced societies—e.g., those following upon urbanization, the growth and decline of particular industries and regions, the aging of population, automation, and the progressively higher levels of skills demanded of the labor force. Some of these same problems appear to have provided an impetus for the development of regional accounting.

This paper seeks to elaborate on the notion of "human resources" in a way that brings it within the purview of those economists concerned with the development of regional accounts. The author is not an economist but a sociologist and demographer with an interest in urban and metropolitan research, and the discussion that follows will inevitably reflect his limited acquaintance with national and regional accounting systems. The emphasis, however, is upon practical matters of measurement and data collection, so that limitations arising out of disciplinary affiliation and background probably pose fewer problems than they might in a paper with a more substantive focus.

1. ACCOUNTING SCHEMES AND THE PROBLEM OF FLOWS

At the national level, there are at least five distinguishable forms of economic account: (1) national income accounts, (2) input-output accounts, (3) flow-of-funds accounts, (4) national balance sheets, and (5) balance-of-payments accounts. Not all of these have regional counterparts, even in theory.[3] As for the meaning of "accounts," we may follow Hoover and Chinitz:

Accounts mean, to us, systematic and quantitative cross-tabulations of economic transactions and claims, primarily in money units and primarily cross-sectional in nature. Basic to this notion of accounts is the feature of double-entry: every transaction and every claim

[3] Richard Ruggles and Nancy D. Ruggles, *National Income Accounts and Income Analysis* (New York: McGraw-Hill Book Co., 2d ed., 1956).

involves two parties, and in principle each item in a set of accounts is cross-checkable because it occurs twice.[4]

Thus one can conceive a series of transactions and claims, comprehending a region, in which various interunit flows are recorded. The "units" or transactors may be legal entities, such as corporations (as in flow-of-funds accounting) or broad sectors, such as whole industries (as in input-output accounts). In any case, transactions are recorded, and usually with reference to changes in stocks by means of a balance sheet.

But what of "social accounts"? Is there an analogous system of double-entry bookkeeping that could be developed to deal with *social* as against economic transactions between units? This is more than a question of simple terminology. Most of the extant discussions of "social accounts" fail to distinguish them from economic accounts and actually focus on problems in economic measurement.[5] It is at this point that one must confront a basic question: Is such an accounting scheme applicable to a population? Can one conceive of a set of interactions or flows between people, viewed as transactors, that is amenable to "accounting" in the sense outlined above? To the best of our knowledge, these issues have been raised only once in the literature on regional accounts. Speaking of the possibilities of intrametropolitan accounting, Harris has pointed out that at least two types of "flow" must be distinguished. "One of these consists of the flows which express regular interaction between elements of the stock. The second consists of those flows which reflect changes in the location of the stock variables—that is, changes in their distribution in space."[6] Only the first of these flows, of course, cor-

[4] Edgar M. Hoover and Benjamin Chinitz, "The Role of Accounts in the Economic Study of the Pittsburgh Metropolitan Region," in *Design of Regional Accounts*, Werner Hochwald, ed. (Baltimore: The Johns Hopkins Press, 1961), pp. 253-54.

[5] See, for example, Charles L. Leven, "A Theory of Regional Social Accounting," in *Papers and Proceedings of the Regional Science Association*, Gerald A. P. Carrothers, ed., 4 (Philadelphia: Regional Science Association, 1958), 221–37. For another effort to outline "a parallel technique to national income accounting . . . for analyzing the social choices made within a population," see Richard L. Meier, "Human Time Allocation: A Basis for Social Accounts," *Journal of the American Institute of Planners*, 35 (Feb. 1959), 27–33.

[6] Britton Harris, "From Intra-metropolitan Conceptual Models to Intrametropolitan Accounts," a paper prepared for the Washington meetings of the Committee on Regional Accounts, Oct. 19-20, 1961, p. 2.

responds to those ordinarily recorded in accounting schemes. But Harris goes one step further: he points out that

> We are dealing not only with economic variables for which the concepts of stocks and flows were invented, but also with demographic and social variables where the application of these concepts is legitimate but perhaps somewhat strained. Thus, for example, we can speak quite freely of a stock of population in a given location at a particular point of time. . . . We can quite clearly speak of changes in location as flows which affect this stock. We can also speak of the flows of goods and people to and from households which constitute the short-term elements of a functioning metropolitan system of interaction. But there is some question in my mind as to what we should call the events of birth and death, marriage and divorce, and separation from the household which also bring about changes in the stock of population in any area over time. These events are flows, but "flows" of a more particular character. Finally, if a population acquires increased income or achieves a higher level of education, the population is no longer the same. Are the events leading to these changes flows? And if so, what is the corresponding stock variable? We may speak of a stock of earning capacity, or a stock of education. But these stocks have many dimensions of the elementary population unit, the individual or household.[7]

It is the main thesis of this paper that the broad concept of "social mobility," as it is conceived in sociology and demography,[8] offers one way out of the rather perplexing situation summarized by Harris, but one that will require a reorientation on the part of economists professing an interest in "social accounts" and "human resources." A secondary thesis is that economists in this field have yet to confront some basic questions relating to the problem of selecting feasible areal units for their work. Again, sociologists and demographers may be helpful in this phase of the total enterprise, especially as their efforts have been directed toward intrametropolitan studies.

[7] *Ibid.*
[8] Some of these ideas are elaborated in Leo F. Schnore, "Social Mobility in Demographic Perspective," *American Sociological Review*, 26 (June 1961), 407–23.

2. TWO MODES OF DATA COLLECTION

When we contemplate the ways in which one might proceed to assess the "stock" of human resources in a given area, together with changes in that stock, it turns out that there are two fundamental modes of measurement that can be employed. As we shall see, the difference between the two methods reduces to a question of timing. Observations may be instantaneous or continuous, i.e., they may be focused on the enumeration of characteristics as of a given point in time or they may be concerned with the recording of events as they occur over time.

We are concerned with means of acquiring information on "human resources"—the quantity and quality of population. Keeping in mind the ineluctable fact of change, we are obliged to take one of two alternatives: (a) an inventory of numbers and characteristics, or (b) a metering of events that give rise to changes in numbers and/or characteristics.[9]

Census Systems. The needs for an inventory are met by a census, i.e., an enumeration of the *number and characteristics* of a given population, whether by a complete count or by a representative sample, as of a given point in time. The static or cross-sectional quality of a census is its fundamental feature, for it provides no more than a "snapshot" of a population and its characteristics. The number of characteristics included is highly variable, ranging from a few simple items to literally dozens of complex features. Theoretically, there is no limit on the number of characteristics subject to enumeration; one could record physical characteristics, possessions, prejudices, and predilections just as readily as the more familiar items found on traditional census schedules.

In the past, the greatest attention shown census materials by economists seems to have been to information regarding manpower and the labor force. More recently, attention has turned to income,

[9] The term "metering" is used here in the sense specified in Harvey S. Perloff, "A National System of Metropolitan Information and Analysis," *American Economic Review*, 52 (May 1962), 356–64.

educational levels, migrant status, and other characteristics. In the accounts framework, the data needs that can be appropriately supplied by a census are easy to exemplify. "We would want to have breakdowns for various characteristics of the labor force (sex, age groupings, race), for skills (i.e., skilled, semiskilled and unskilled), and for major occupational groupings." [10] Such items, of course, are commonly enumerated in all modern census systems, whether they involve a complete enumeration or depend upon sampling methods.

Registration Systems. In contrast, the needs for metering are more appropriately met by a system of registration, i.e., a comprehensive and continuous recording and compilation of *events* in a particular population, at or near their times of occurrence. Here the static or cross-sectional character of a census is lacking; in fact, it is precisely the dynamic quality of registration that is its most fundamental feature. The "snapshot" provided by a census is augmented by a "moving picture" of closely spaced observations. The events subject to registration are also variable in the extreme. We tend to think of registration systems as limited to so-called "vital events," such as births and deaths. In actuality, a very large number of changes in status are amenable to registration. For almost every characteristic that can be enumerated in a census, there is a comparable change that can be observed and recorded in a registration system.

Events that are theoretically amenable to registration include migration (changes in place of residence) and various types of "social mobility" (changes in status). Movements between modern nation-states, or "international migrations," are commonly registered. In contrast, "internal migration," or change of residence within a country, is less frequently a subject of registration. As a mode of observation and measurement, registration is also logically applicable to other types of mobility, in the sense of movements within the socioeconomic system, or status changes. Thus occupational changes may be recorded in a registration system; they are analogous to changes in, say, marital status, and they may be registered just like marriages and divorces, albeit at greater expense.

[10] Harvey S. Perloff, "Relative Regional Economic Growth: An Approach to Regional Accounts," in Hochwald, *op. cit.*, p. 63.

In any case, these two basic modes of data collection—census and registration systems—must be seen as complementary devices. They are particularly informative when their products are combined, as in the construction of series of vital rates.[11] Each provides information that is not directly derivable from the other, although it is important to realize that a census may provide surrogate data on migration and mobility. Thus Bogue describes "mobility statistics," census data referring to a "change in some status during an arbitrarily selected interval of time," and "tenure statistics," wherein "each person is asked when he entered his present status."[12] The 1960 Census of Population of the United States contained two questions on migration and residential mobility that took these forms: individuals in the 25-per-cent sample were asked (a) where they lived in 1955, and (b) the date at which they moved into their present housing unit.

If one assumes the continuous and efficient operation of a registration system over a number of decades, the need for a census practically disappears, except as an independent means of checking the registration system. One simply stops the system at an arbitrarily chosen point in time and counts the number of persons with each characteristic of interest as of that date. In effect, this is the "census" method commonly employed in Sweden, which (like a few other countries) has had a continuous registration system in operation for a great many years. "With these systems of accounting, a balance sheet can be drawn at any point of time indicating the status and characteristics of the residents of any area, a periodic summary of changes in status can be prepared (persons reaching school age, voting age, pension age, etc.), the rate and direction of migration readily determined, and the factors producing movement in the population readily evaluated."[13] It is important to note the similar-

[11] The combination is not easy once the analyst gets beyond the simplest types of inquiry. See Philip M. Hauser and Evelyn M. Kitagawa, "Social and Economic Mortality Differentials in the United States, 1960: Outline of a Research Project," *1960 Proceedings of the Social Statistics Section, American Statistical Association* (Washington: American Statistical Association, 1960), pp. 116–20.
[12] Donald J. Bogue, "The Quantitative Study of Social Dynamics and Social Change," *American Journal of Sociology*, 57 (May 1952), 565–68.
[13] Dorothy S. Thomas, "The Continuous Register System of Population Accounting," in National Resources Committee, *The Problems of a Changing Population* (Washington, 1938), App. C, p. 276.

ity between this method, applied to actual populations, and the "census" of a simulated socioeconomic system.[14]

It would appear that economists concerned with the development of genuine "social accounts," whether on a national or a regional basis, would do well to consider the possibilities of instituting a full-scale system of continuous registration. In the United States, of course, such a system is lacking and probably not feasible, because of administrative problems and sheer cost considerations. What we have, in effect, is a large number of partial registration systems, covering only selected portions of the total population, systems that at present are altogether lacking in integration. Moreover, only one exploratory effort has been directed toward making use of the partial data in answering analytical questions; Bogue has attempted to make use of Bureau of Old Age and Survivors Insurance data to get at the relations between migration and labor mobility.[15]

If the goals are to quantify the stock of "human resources" and to assess changes in that stock, procedures must be devised that will yield not only "snapshots" of the population as of particular points in time but also "moving pictures" of significant changes within the population. In the field of regional accounts, one is struck with the apparent lack of consensus concerning the relevant characteristics of population on which data are needed. An exploration of the literature, however, does yield a rough order of priorities. At the very least, one can discern some degree of agreement on a few items of information for which widespread demand is evident. The following section takes up two of these items.

3. TWO CENTRAL PROBLEMS

Hirsch has identified a large number of personal characteristics for which regional data are desirable; these include "about twenty

---

[14] Guy H. Orcutt, "Microanalytic Models for Regional Analysis," in Hochwald, *op. cit.*, esp. p. 245.

[15] Donald J. Bogue, *An Exploratory Study of Migration and Labor Mobility Using Social Security Data*, Studies in Population Distribution, No. 1 (Oxford, Ohio: Scripps Foundation for Research in Population Problems, 1950). Problems involved in developing a full-scale registration system are discussed in Halbert L. Dunn, "A National Identity Registration System to Synthesize Social Statistics," *Estadistica*, 11 (Sept. 1953), 605–15.

Demographic Data, forty-six Economic Data, six Education Data, five Health Data, three Welfare Data, and five Law Enforcement Data." [16] This is, by all odds, the most comprehensive and ambitious listing of desiderata in the literature. Hirsch wants everything. Elsewhere, one gets the impression that most scholars concerned with regional accounts would be satisfied with far less information; in particular, data on migration and various kinds of mobility seem to be the most pressing needs. Perloff has expressed this desire in summary fashion: "Systematized record keeping on stocks as well as flows is a vital need. . . . Equally important is an inventory of the human assets: what kinds of people are in the community, what kinds are coming in, and what kinds are leaving." [17] In our society, it appears that so-called "structural" unemployment is coming to receive more attention than the "cyclical" unemployment that preoccupied Keynes. Indeed, the identification and measurement of various kinds of labor mobility and immobility—whether occupational, industrial, or geographic—might come to be regarded as tasks more critical than those of assessing the movement of major Keynesian variables, such as investment and consumption. In any case, the movement of people within the socioeconomic system would appear to warrant the closest attention by regional accountants.

Migration. The demographic and sociological literature on this subject is so vast that one would be ill-advised to attempt a summary or overview of even the methodological portion of it. It is sufficient for present purposes to note that the absence of a registration system in the United States has resulted in a literature that is overwhelmingly concerned with methods of estimation and measurement. Numbers of migrants, gross and net, can be estimated with some degree of confidence, but the study of characteristics of migrants lags far behind, particularly as different forms of selectivity may operate in different types of migrant streams. (People flowing from rural to urban areas differ from those making up the city-suburban stream, etc.) From the standpoint of regional accounts,

---

[16] Werner Z. Hirsch, "Design and Use of Regional Accounts," *American Economic Review*, 52 (May 1962), 372–73.

[17] "A National System of Metropolitan Information and Analysis," *op. cit.*, p. 361.

this is particularly distressing, because the interest lies in the kind of people entering and leaving different areas.

Perhaps those economists who are vitally concerned with regional accounts would do well to prepare an illustrative list of those features of migration in which they are most interested. Such a list would also serve to give some focus to the efforts of those in the demographic fraternity who are concerned with the measurement of migration. It may turn out that some of the problems which seem so formidable at first glance are not really so troublesome. For example, most "migration" covers a very short distance; if it should turn out that the student of regional accounts has little need for information on *intra*regional movement, the problems may be far less imposing than otherwise.[18] In the course of developing such a list, it would also be highly desirable to have a specification of the areal units for which data are desired. (This is a problem to which we shall turn below.)

Mobility. We use the term "social mobility" in a broad and generic sense, to refer to changes in individual status within the context of a socioeconomic system. Thus changes in marital status, job transfers, and the acquisition of further education are all conceived as forms of social mobility. Such movements or status changes differ in type, for example, according to whether or not the change is reversible in direction. Thus the acquisition of another increment of formal schooling makes for an irreversible change of educational status; in contrast, one may leave a job for another and subsequently return to his earlier occupation.

Again, it would be most helpful to demographers and sociologists who are interested in the subject of social mobility to have a list of priorities from those economists who are concerned with the development of regional accounts. Our impression is that educational mobility is the form that would attract the greatest amount of interest at this time, especially as the broad concept of human re-

---

[18] ". . . while our concern is with interstate migration, we recognize that the major part of population mobility in the past has been related to migration into metropolitan areas and suburbs." Louis Delwart and Sidney Sonenblum, "Regional Account Projections in the Context of National Projections," in Hochwald, *op. cit.*, p. 206.

sources has infiltrated the field and as public concern with the level of skills in the population has been so widely expressed. Without an actual promise of immediately applicable results, it must be said that there is a growing body of sociological research that is focused on questions of the educational status and aspirations of various segments of the population, and some of this material also bears on the question of migratory behavior in relation to other kinds of mobility.[19]

4. THE PROBLEM OF AREAL UNITS

In all the foregoing discussion, we have avoided an issue that is of fundamental importance, i.e., the question of areal units. It is only in connection with our brief treatment of migration that we have made any allusion to this matter. Perhaps it is so basic an issue that it is likely to be overlooked. To state it most baldly: What are the "regions" for which "regional accounts" are to be developed?

Hochwald has pointed out that "the very definition of the region offers many ambiguities. Its size may vary from the small neighborhood within a larger metropolitan area to the huge subregion within a continent."[20] Each type of unit seems to have its advocates. Thus Delwart and Sonenblum see the state as "the best compromise region" for their purposes.[21] Others speak on behalf of the metropolitan area as the unit of primary interest. Still others apparently have in mind very large regions, such as "the South."

Some useful guidelines have been offered by Richard and Nancy Ruggles:

There are two characteristics that can be used to define meaningful geographical areas. First, one may be interested in a specific geographic area because it conforms to a *political* subdivision. . . . Second, a region may be defined in *economic* terms, containing sev-

[19] See, for example, Ronald Freedman and Deborah Freedman, "Farm-Reared Elements in the Nonfarm Population," *Rural Sociology*, 21 (March 1956), 50–61. They show that rural-to-urban migrants in the United States have tended to enter the urban class structure at or near the bottom of the scale, whether their status is measured by income, occupation, or education.
[20] In Hochwald, *op. cit.*, p. xiv.
[21] *Ibid.*, p. 201.

veral political units which are bound together by their common economic interest. . . . There is no ready answer to what the smallest regional unit should be. Political and economic criteria may, in many cases, lead to entirely different regional breakdowns. In any case, it seems reasonable to aim for breakdowns by states and local political subdivisions, and in addition by important metropolitan areas."[22]

Still another important consideration has been introduced by Burkhead. In discussing Perloff's recommendations, he notes that "After we have arrived at the point when the Perloff prescription has been filled, we will find that there is no regional public or private authority with area-wide competence for decision-making. Indeed, there is no region that may be commonly defined for a wide range of problems."[23] This raises an issue that hinges on the extent to which regional accounting is to be developed for *policy* purposes. Ideally, the region should be an actual or potential decision unit. Thus it might be a political unit (e.g., a state) over which a common system of authority has been established, and for which there exists a relevant audience of decision-makers. At a more gross level, the Federal Reserve District might be an appropriate regional unit.[24] At a lower level, the metropolitan region might be a suitable unit, at least in those areas where some degree of regional consciousness has been manifested in area-wide authorities or planning organizations. Certainly there must be some appropriate audience of policy-makers if one of Perloff's prescriptions is to be realized; as he has held, "a metropolis would do well to provide for the preparation of an annual 'state-of-the-region' report which would present the key data and analyze their implications, somewhat in the manner of the state-of-the-Union message presented by the President."[25] Alongside this request we must consider the opinion advanced by two experienced students of the metropolitan region, Hoover and Chinitz: "It may be remarked in passing that any systematic effort to deal with the internal spatial pattern in terms of accounts seems

[22] *Ibid.*, pp. 124–25; italics added.
[23] *Ibid.*, p. 67.
[24] Joseph L. Fisher, "Potential Contributions of Regional Science to the Field of Economics," in *Papers and Proceedings of the Regional Science Association*, Gerald A. P. Carrothers and William Alonso, eds., 3 (Philadelphia: Regional Science Association, 1957), 17–23.
[25] Perloff, "A National System of Metropolitan Information and Analysis," *American Economic Review*, 52 (May 1962), 361–62.

wholly unfeasible."[26] If an outsider may make one last recommendation, it is that economists concerned with the development of regional accounts undertake some "feasibility studies" concerning the regional units to be employed. The present availability of data should probably bulk large in such deliberations.[27]

If the notion of intrametropolitan accounts is actually a will-o'-the-wisp, it would certainly be better to know it soon. If the metropolitan region does turn out to be a manageable unit for accounting purposes, however, economists might do well to look into the work that has been done by those sociologists who are concerned with the internal spatial structure and dynamics of the metropolis. The economist's principal interest in intrametropolitan accounts is linked to questions of local public finance: Where are the "resources" and where are the "needs"? Although they pose their queries in different ways, sociologists are producing data that are admirably suited to answering some of the economist's questions. At the minimum, new questions are raised.[28]

5. CONCLUSIONS

It might appear that the interest of American economists in the quantity and quality of population was revived only with the discovery of the "underdeveloped" area.[29] A comparable development

---

[26] In Hochwald, *op. cit.*, p. 262.

[27] See the *Inventory of Federal Statistics for Standard Metropolitan Statistical Areas, Counties, and Cities* (Washington: Bureau of the Budget, Executive Office of the President, Jan. 1961). In addition, the new *Statistical Abstract of the United States, 1962* (Washington: U.S. Bureau of the Census) contains a detailed "Guide to State Statistical Abstracts."

[28] For a guide to the relevant sociological literature, see Leo F. Schnore, "The Socio-economic Status of Cities and Suburbs," *American Sociological Review*, 28 (Feb. 1963), 76–85. The enormous potential of true registration data for intrametropolitan research is demonstrated in Sidney Goldstein, "Some Economic Consequences of Suburbanization in the Copenhagen Metropolitan Area," *American Journal of Sociology*, 68 (March 1963), 551–64.

[29] Harvey Leibenstein, *Economic Backwardness and Economic Growth* (New York: John C. Wiley & Sons, 1957); Ansley J. Coale and Edgar M. Hoover, *Population Growth and Economic Development in Low-Income Countries* (Princeton: Princeton University Press, 1958); Vincent Heath Whitney, "Population in Theories of Economic Development," in *International Population Conference*, Louis Henry and Wilhelm Winkler, eds. (Vienna: International Union for the Scientific Study of Population, 1959), pp. 149–57.

on the domestic front seems to be well under way, if one may judge from the recent emphasis upon human resources in the economic literature. The newly developing field of regional accounts appears to share this interest in demographic matters, and it should, but it has yet to confront some fundamental questions of feasibility and to establish priorities with respect to data needs. While they can provide no ready-made answers, many sociologists and demographers are working on related problems, and they stand ready to serve in clarifying some of the basic questions.

COMMENT

HAL H. WINSBOROUGH
Duke University

In discussing the measurement of human resources in a regional-accounting framework, Schnore points to two major problems. The first has to do with the collection of data; the second with problems in the definition of regions.

In discussing the availability of information on human resources, Schnore notes that data are usually collected in two ways: by a census or by a registration system. Since the basic problem in human-resources accounting is that of flows, i.e., of mobility and migration, Schnore focuses on the potentialities of the registration system. He builds a strong case that progress toward a satisfactory system of accounts would be considerably speeded by the development of a full-scale system of continuous registration.

If the development of a system of human-resources accounting were dependent on the institution of such a registration system, however, it seems likely that it would be postponed for a long time. In the face of a sometimes recalcitrant populace, it is difficult enough to operate a census, for which there is a constitutional provision. The institution of a nationwide registration of vital events alone required a long battle only relatively recently won. The notion of extending registration to changes in job, changes in residence, and so on is awesome indeed. Recognizing this difficulty, Schnore suggests a beginning be made through the comparison and codification of records from existing partial registration systems. This writer knows of fairly little experience with this procedure. The greater bulk of the experience has been with the comparison of census records and those of certain registration systems. Perhaps some discussion of this experience will clarify some of the problems involved in the comparison and codification process.

Following the 1950 Census, a post-enumeration survey was conducted to estimate errors in census procedure.[1] A part of the analysis of this survey entailed a record check of individuals' responses on both the census and the post-enumeration survey against records from other agencies. For sub-samples of the post-enumeration-survey sample, responses were matched against birth certificates, Social Security records, Veterans Administration records, Immigration and Naturalization Service records, and Internal Revenue Service records of federal income-tax returns. These matchings proved quite difficult. In all the studies there was a substantial residue of cases where the matching records could not be found or could not be definitely identified as relating to the same person.

In spite of the difficulties involved in matching records and census returns, the procedure was thought fruitful enough to warrant further investigation. At least one large-scale matching study is currently nearing completion in which procedures to reduce error and bias from non-matching records have been introduced.[2]

This experience in matching records of registration systems and census returns points to what would probably be the largest problem in organizing existing partial registration systems: figuring out who is who. Perhaps a first step in the codification of existing partial registration systems, then, might be an attack on this problem

---

[1] U.S. Bureau of the Census, *The Post Enumeration Survey: 1950*, Bureau of the Census Technical Paper No. 4 (Washington, 1960).

[2] See Philip M. Hauser and Evelyn M. Kitagawa, "Social and Economic Mortality Differentials in the United States, 1960: Outline of a Research Project," *1960 Proceedings of the Social Statistics Section, American Statistical Association* (Washington: American Statistical Association, 1960), pp. 116–20.

through the development of a set of general identifying numbers for members of the population. The Internal Revenue Service is currently instituting the use of social-security numbers as identifying numbers for all persons returning an income-tax form. If the use of social-security numbers as identifying numbers were to become universal, it would make the chore of matching records among agencies much less costly and less subject to error. Within agencies, too, the use of identifying numbers would make possible a reliable matching of records.

This observation brings up an additional source of information on mobility and migration which is ignored by Schnore. The information currently collected by the Bureau of the Census could, if properly compiled, provide excellent data about mobility and migration. If it were possible to compare returns of persons for two or more censuses, it would be possible to determine the number of persons who, in the intervening period, had moved from one location to another, changed occupations, changed marital status, changed the industry in which they work, etc. Furthermore, given such collated information, it would be possible to find out, for persons mobile in one census characteristic, their status in any other characteristic both before and after the transition. In other words, given such collated information, a matrix of transition could be prepared for any characteristic or set of joint characteristics. Such matrices are amenable to fairly sophisticated analysis, particularly if tables over several time lapses are available.[3]

The Bureau of the Census has, apparently, had some experience in matching records between censuses. In the previously mentioned post-enumeration survey, some attempt was made to match returns against 1920 Census records. As I understand it, such matching currently requires that the respondent not only know his address at the time of the earlier census but also know who was listed as head of the household under which he was enumerated. To expect such information after thirty years seems somewhat unreasonable. Over a shorter period, however, it might lead to less difficulty.

[3] See, e.g., Isadore Blumen, Marvin Koyan, Philip J. McCarthy, *The Industrial Mobility of the Labor Force as a Probability Process* (Ithaca, N.Y.: Cornell University, 1955); and Leo A. Goodman, "Statistical Methods for the Mover-Stayer Model," *Journal of the American Statistical Association,* 56 (1961), 841–68.

These observations suggest that economists trying to devise a system of human-resources accounts may be able to anticipate that within several decades information will be available on the ten-year mobility of the population. Within any one region, one would think, a series of such tables would be useful tools in decision-making.

For more immediate use, a modification of this procedure might be devised. If, a year or two following a census, a sample survey were conducted which, in addition to collecting the required replication of census data, asked place of residence and head of the household as of the census date, a satisfactory matching might be possible. This proposed method of collecting information has many difficulties, of course. At minimum, however, it would provide more information about joint effects of mobility and migration than has heretofore been available. Such a survey could be conducted on a regional basis as well as on a national one.

This discussion, then, suggests there is a real possibility of getting information about both mobility and migration of a kind never before available in this country. The use of high-speed electronic computers for processing data, combined with a policy decision to extend social-security numbers to become general identifying numbers, would make possible the codification of existing records. Experience already gained in matching records suggests the possibility of getting a reasonable amount of information even under current systems of identification. This possibility presents an exciting prospect for students of human resources.

The second basic issue raised by Schnore is that of the definition of regions. Of this problem Schnore says: ". . . economists in this field have yet to confront some basic questions relating to the problem of selecting feasible areal units for their work. Again, sociologists and demographers may be helpful in this phase of the total enterprise, especially as their efforts have been directed toward intrametropolitan studies."

Since the author of this discussion is a sociologist and demographer, as Schnore is, he, of course, agrees with this statement. For those less committed to the utility of the sociological and demographic disciplines as applied to the problem of definition of regions, however, perhaps an illustration is in order.

In considering strategy in the analysis of regions, many economists seem to regard the delineation of regions as a separate problem from the investigation of intraregional and interregional relationships. Thus, one has the impression that many economists would agree with Isard and Reiner that "The empirical delimitation of the regional system of reference is an indispensable task which geographers must perform to provide basic material for not only regional scientists but for all scientists." [4]

Sociologists, however, dealing with the metropolitan region, or the metropolitan community as they sometimes prefer to call it, have developed a way of thinking about the problem which contradicts the utility of this rigid division of labor. In a recent investigation, for instance, Pappenfort holds:

A "community"—whether the concept is applied to plants, animals, or human beings and their institutions—by definition is not a discrete entity. It is an identifiable set of symbiotic relationships which necessarily are involved with and have implications for other such identifiable sets. Several or many such communities constitute an ecological "field" which is the fundamental unit of analysis. Hypotheses and methods used in the study of several communities or even a single community need to be predicated upon a process of abstraction from the more inclusive area.[5]

The implications of this formulation of the problem seem clear. If the delineation of a region implies the description of an identifiable set of relationships which can reasonably be abstracted from the whole of the "field," then the investigation of intra- and inter-"regional" relationships must go hand-in-hand with the process of delineation. This, then, seems a basic contribution made by the sociological and demographic experience with metropolitan studies: that the delineation of reasonable areas, the investigation of intra- and inter-area relationships, and the development of useful data are all three intertwined in the process of investigating the areal aspects of the social system.

[4] "Summary Paper," *1961 Papers & Proceedings of the Regional Science Association*, Vol. VIII.

[5] Donnell M. Pappenfort, "The Ecological Field and the Metropolitan Community: Manufacturing and Management," *American Journal of Sociology*, 64 (Jan. 1959), 380–85.

MANPOWER MOVEMENTS: A PROPOSED APPROACH TO MEASUREMENT

GEORGE J. STOLNITZ
Indiana University

This brief paper is based on the premise that movement of commodities between areas and industries, although rightly a core focus of regional analysis, has usurped too large a part of the input-output approach. Imaginative thinking needs to be applied to other aspects of the process of relative regional growth or decline. Probably no less important than commodity flows are the corresponding movements of manpower, regarded both as response to new job opportunities and as a determinant of demand, thereby further shaping the nature of such opportunities.

Specifically, the comments here center about the suggestion that "from-to" tables for manpower need to be developed, along lines more or less analogous to those of regional input-output models for commodities. The basic flow variables would be movements of the labor force between initial industrial (or occupational) status and region and eventual status and region, between the beginning and end of a given period. "Inputs" in this sense denote the amounts of manpower provided each employing sector by various sources of supply, where these are distinguished by their origin rather than the nature of their productive contribution. "Outputs" denote the uses, by regional and industrial destination, of a given source of supply. The element of formal analogy with conventional input-output becomes closer beyond this definitional point. Thus numbers can be changed to coefficients and a "final bill" of demand by manpower can be converted through matrix inversion into a set of supplies by origin. In a constantly adjusting labor market, interdependence frequently arises in the form of two-way or multilateral shifts from area to area and industry to industry.

The resulting tabulations would provide, for the first time, an integrated view of the manpower component of interregional relations. Regional research has done relatively little in this area, beyond confirming its importance. It is true that we know a good deal about migration and changing industrial composition. But we know—or have done—almost nothing about the cross-classifications between the two and nothing about the connections between regional-industrial origins and the corresponding destinations. Documentation along the lines suggested here could help fill much of these gaps. It would provide novel information on the process of labor-force responses in the face of shifting job opportunities, the speed of such responses, the degree and influence of intervening opportunities as part of the process, and the mobility propensities of the various regional-industrial components of the labor force. Much of its prospective usefulness would stem from the fact that the data would be oriented to the actual movements of individuals, rather than before-after comparisons between groups. Tying in the personal and household characteristics of individuals with their mobility experience would, in turn, illuminate the feedback relations likely to hold between the changing employment pattern of a region and its growth. To cite only one example, inclusion of an origins-destination question in the Census would permit direct identification of housing characteristics for each cell in the from-to matrix. An especially significant facet of the interplay between the build-up of a region's export industries and its residentiary activities could thereby be explored in ways not previously possible.

1. THE PROPOSAL

The from-to tables just outlined would in effect be cross-classifications of region and industry (or occupation) at the end of any given study period on the columns axis—the "using" sectors, and the corresponding cross-classifications at the beginning of the period on the rows axis—the "supplying" sectors. Aggregate controls would be provided by the total employed or total labor force at either the beginning or the end of the period, e.g., as provided by a census.

Transformation of numbers to ratios would be on the basis of column totals. To repeat, the coefficients represent manpower-origin parameters, the regional-industrial (or occupational) contributions to the end-period labor force. Column totals correspond to the labor-input row of the ordinary input-output table.

The specific definitions of units to be employed—for example, the length of the study period—or the choice of regions could be determined only by practice and application and in the light of data availability. Nevertheless, some general comments would seem indicated here.

The length of the study period should probably be in excess of a year, perhaps as much as five years. Unlike commodities, whose movements in a year are typically sufficient for meeting the problem of sampling in time, population and manpower are likely to move more slowly and unstably in the short run. Experience with migration data suggests that an adequately large body of numbers is compiled only over periods of several years, when interest centers on small population categories. In the present case, of manpower subclassified by both industry and region, much the same conclusion can be anticipated. Obviously, there would be no harm in a series of short-term tables, since these could be combined and netted out as deemed advisable. It is well to keep in mind, however, that adequately reliable data might first become available after a sequence of compilations.

The choice of regions would affect the usefulness of the proposed tables for investigating feedback relations between industrial structure and residentiary activities. Shifts between industries or occupations without any spatial resettlement, for example, typically have lesser impact on consumption patterns and public investment than do shifts involving spatial movements. Accordingly, a sufficiently fine regional breakdown may be provided by units large enough to minimize the effects of intraregional job commuting.

Combinations of counties might be the answer in this respect. Regional research offers few functional guidelines for making judgments, being much more agreed on the need for studying regions than on their optimal selection for either study or policy. Presumably the choice of units would be settled by trial and error or convenience in any event.

Trial and error would also be required to determine a choice between occupation or industry. The former would appear more useful for exhibiting individual propensities, by linking past training and job experience with present jobs more closely than does an industry classification. I would also anticipate that data obtained from interview surveys of individuals and households would be more accurately reported by occupation, particularly with respect to status in an earlier period. On the other hand, an industrial classification would be much more closely linked with the data and data systems most prominent in regional analysis, such as movements of commodities, location of firms, and composition of final demand. For this reason I am tentatively but not weakly persuaded that at least the first major efforts to construct manpower from-to tables should be couched in industrial terms. The occupational implications of such movements could be ascertained if desired by means of "side models," involving occupational classification within industries by region. The use of complementary models is customary by now in input-output work and would appear to raise no special problems in the present instance.

A much greater potential complication is that the classifications typically demanded of manpower tend to be more fine than those for goods and services. Thus, age, sex, and color are staple if not indispensable categories in all demographic-economic investigations, with no counterparts in commodity analysis. The distributions of interregional or interindustrial movements by these characteristics are often highly skewed. The younger worker is more likely to make an interstate move in changing jobs than the older one; sex distribution is often highly uneven by type of industry; non-white workers are typically far more concentrated in some industries over others than are white workers. Aggregation over these variables might therefore conceal a good deal that should be made explicit. On the one hand, even with stable from-to coefficients within each demographic category, changing demographic composition could lead to variable aggregate coefficients. On the other hand, stable aggregate coefficients may be inadequate for a great many of the uses which might be made of the from-to compilations. In predicting recruitment patterns or their consequences for regional demand, it may make a good deal of difference whether the shift is made by white or non-white workers.

Although it would be comforting here to fall back on the usual disclaimer in the input-output literature, that the prospective stability or instability of the coefficients is an "empirical" question, it would be more reassuring if the question had an answer. Fortunately, answers should be obtainable from a variety of sources. Any future Bureau of the Census compilation that could be used to fill out an aggregate from-to table would almost certainly also provide age-sex-color information for the various cells. Hence disaggregated multiple tables should be available. If the resulting disaggregated coefficients were found to have appropriate stability properties, the final demand for labor by each employing industry and region (columns) could be broken down first by demographic categories and the coefficients applied to predict its origins by source of supply. Conversely, if the aggregate coefficients proved more stable, origins by supplying sectors could be obtained first and demographic breakdowns subsequently by side investigations.

Another question to be settled is whether the manpower universe under study should be defined according to its beginning-period composition and traced forward in time or should be defined by the end-period composition and traced backward. In principle either system could be employed, according to purpose. The differences between the two totals on a national basis would involve accessions and separations because of retirement, mortality, new workers, change in the net unemployed and net shifts into or out of the labor force of such other categories as secondary workers. Again, various approaches might be employed with respect to each of these.

Thus retirement could be included explicitly under a household column, corresponding to the household sector in the original closed Leontief model. Alternatively, the retired could be ignored as not belonging to the employed labor force at the end of the study period.

The manner in which the retired could be identified, if at all, would obviously depend upon the nature and purpose of the data-collection procedures utilized to fill out the matrix. An end-period collection system involving the employed would automatically exclude the retired. A "forward-looking" system starting at the beginning of the period would automatically include them.

It is easy to envisage major areas of research interest in which the retired could be ignored, though the opposite instances probably come to mind more readily. In addition to the fact that there is an interest in this category for its own sake, the tendency is to think of a national labor force and its projected redistribution in the future, including moves to retirement. Yet quite a different orientation may be relevant and have equally important purposes. Thus suppose we are given, in standard input-output fashion, a projected "final bill of manpower," yielding the column totals of the proposed tables. The predictive use of the tables would then be focused on the origins of those assumed to be employed at a specified later date, irrespective of those who had left the labor force in the interim.

Similar considerations would apply to separations from the labor force because of mortality or because of returns to household status by housewives and secondary workers in general.

Nevertheless it is simpler to assume, as will be done here, that there is a household column to include all separations from the labor force. Useful and reliable estimates of separations should not be difficult to obtain. Moreover, inclusion of a household column would have the desirable property of balancing a corresponding household row, which is needed to take care of labor-force accessions, particularly new workers.

The unemployed could be handled by a separate row and column or included with the household row and column as desired or as the data permit. The main question here with respect to separate documentation is whether reliable information could be obtained for persons unemployed as of the beginning of the study period, particularly if the period is of several years' duration. Also, the numbers might become small and erratic under a fairly fine classification of regions and industries. As with many analogous questions raised here, the issue could best be settled in a specific context.

Another general question, which is transverse to the ones already considered, is whether the movements should be gross or net. Gross data on a comprehensive, forward-looking basis could be obtained only by continuous registration, and hence can be ignored for the United States. An adequate substitute would be provided by compilations of end-period data on recent work histories, documented by place-of-work and industrial classifications. Such histories would be analogous to the survey designs used by the Bureau of the Census to obtain reproductive histories of women. Net data, in contrast, would entail a much lesser statistical burden on the collecting agencies and might therefore be a preferable starting point. In this case the flow statistics on movements would really represent differences between stocks; the universe would be defined by end-period manpower (with or without inclusion of a household column) and cross-classified by initial-period status. Here as elsewhere, the choice may not be between black and white over the longer run. Net data could be supplemented by occasional inquiries on gross movements and by longitudinal studies of the kind being increasingly undertaken by private and public research groups.

2. DATA SOURCES

Statistical patchwork and improvisation have been typical of input-output research throughout its history. The research area proposed here would no doubt be similarly vulnerable, whatever the compromises on disaggregation and however convenient the definitions adopted for empirical work. Fortunately, the prospects for documenting manpower movements start with a considerable advantage in terms of prospective linkages with existing data systems. The Decennial Census already asks for residence as of a given earlier date, showing city or town for those who have moved. The 1950 Census asked for residence a year earlier. The 1960 Census shifted to residence five years earlier, in order to compile a larger body of migration experience than would have been obtainable over the shorter period. Occupation and industry are also given for persons answering the migration question, and it seems safe to predict that much the same questions on all these items will be repeated in 1970.

All that would be needed to open the door to implementing the present proposal would be an added question concerning industry and region of employment as of an earlier date. No doubt such additions are more readily envisaged than accepted, since the Bureau of the Census is deluged by requests for questions on the Census and can select only a few. Nevertheless there is reason to be hopeful that the needed information could in fact be obtained, if the research being suggested were to make substantial progress before 1970 Census decisions are reached.

Meanwhile, or even alternatively, a good deal can be done by means of the Bureau's Current Population Survey (CPS), particularly if its sample size were increased in the next few years. In this connection, it is worth emphasizing that the recent President's Committee to Appraise Employment and Unemployment Statistics suggested that the CPS sample be expanded to "perhaps of the order of ten times its present size" within the next decade and that such expansion "should be started promptly." [1]

It is by now standard practice for the Bureau to incorporate special topics into the CPS which vary from month to month. Indeed, it happens that a survey on the work history of the longer-run unemployed over a period of about five years is scheduled for just about the time of this writing. Similar surveys, but for all members of the labor force and asking information on region of previous work, could provide a beginning point for analysis in relatively short order, long before 1970. Such information could be readily tied in with the long-established program by the Bureau to survey migration on a recurring basis (a problem here would

---

[1] President's Committee to Appraise Employment and Unemployment Statistics, *Measuring Employment and Unemployment* (Washington, 1962), p. 150.

be to reconcile time periods, since the migration data cover a year only).

The main drawback in the CPS is its small sample size. Until now the Bureau has been unwilling to give geographical detail for anything smaller than major regions and has shown no cross-classifications with industry. The reason clearly is that a breakdown of the CPS materials by industries and regions would often lead to highly unstable numbers.

But even if sample size of the CPS stayed unchanged in the next few years, a useful start could be made on subsequent data needs with small surveys and experience could be accumulated. Should the advice of the President's Committee be heeded in the near future, the prospects for availability of reliable data would be commensurately advanced.

Sources beyond these are much more fragmentary or indirect. Nevertheless, there are such sources, which should be carefully explored. The Bureau of Labor Statistics monthly series on employment by industries, which is based on a monthly sample of 180,000 establishments, could provide a good deal of detail, largely unpublished to date, on non-farm employment by place of work and industry. Information from the CPS series and the last Census on regional movements of persons classified by end-period industry could be applied, under simplifying—or heroic—assumptions, to the observed differences in BLS data between beginning-period and end-period numbers in the various from-to cells. Similarly, such information could be applied to the 1950 and 1960 Censuses to obtain alternative estimates of from-to values. This procedure would have the advantage of yielding more refined classifications by regions or industries but also the disadvantages of netting out a longer period and allowing a greater margin of error in the methodology.

Still another potential source for initial research is the Social Security Administration records system, which provides sequential information on place of work and name of employer of the covered population. Samples of the records could be used in collecting work histories, complemented by mail or field survey as needed to determine information not given directly. The cost of such surveys would probably be small. At least some of the categories of manpower not covered could be estimated roughly from other records; for example, the agricultural labor force could be estimated from Department of Agriculture compilations.

Finally and at least for the sake of completeness, it may be noted that a variety of longitudinal or follow-up surveys exist, which are often undertaken for quite different purposes, such as health research, but which could be utilized or expanded to include labor-force questions.

3. SUMMARY

To sum up, although statistical materials for filling out a manpower from-to matrix do not yet exist in any finished form, they are closely akin, and can be readily added, to ongoing data systems in the government. Possibly, a first full-blown compilation might have to await the 1970 Census. On the other hand there is no need to wait this long before initiating work in the area, in view of the existence and promise of a substantial number of alternatives to the Census. Assuming the underlying idea presented here is warranted, there should be ample room for implementing it in the next several years.

TOWARD AN INTEGRATED SYSTEM OF REGIONAL ACCOUNTS: STOCKS, FLOWS, AND THE ANALYSIS OF THE PUBLIC SECTOR

HARVEY S. PERLOFF [1] and CHARLES L. LEVEN [1]

Committee of Nine, Alliance for Progress; and Resources for the Future, Inc.

University of Pittsburgh

It is generally accepted that a system of regional accounts should be helpful in at least three ways. It should provide a useful base of information for decision-making by both public and private units in urban communities. It should help in the evaluation of the regional impact of national policies and activities, as with regard to spending, tariff changes, and the like. It should contribute to a deeper understanding of our urban regions and to the fuller development of a theory of regional change.

Several of the papers given at the first Conference on Regional Accounts [2] made the point that to achieve objectives such as these, a system of regional accounts must incorporate data on stocks (assets) as well as on flows, that information on stock-flow and flow-stock relationships is essential for most types of dynamic regional analyses.[3] While some general suggestions were made con-

---

[1] We have made a number of changes in our paper in line with suggestions provided by Werner Hirsch. We are grateful to him for his highly constructive and valuable comments on our original manuscript.

[2] Published in *Design of Regional Accounts*, Werner Hochwald, ed. (Baltimore: The Johns Hopkins Press, 1961).

[3] By stock-flow relationships we mean the increase in flows (at equilibrium or capacity) that would result from a given increase in stocks. For individual firms or industries these would be partial production functions; for more aggregated sectors they would be capital-output ratios. Flow-stock relation-

cerning such information, the subject was not carried very far. In this paper, we attempt to go some distance further and outline a suggested scheme for an expanded regional-accounts system within which stocks and flows can be treated in an integrated fashion and within which the analysis of structural change itself can be made a part of the model. We are only too aware of the fact that what we present is a rather primitive and still quite partial scheme. Our hope, however, is that the suggested approach can prove to be fruitful, i.e., that it provides a useful base for extension and refinement.

One does not tackle the subject of stocks and stock-flow relationships very lightly; it is a field well known for its endless difficulties, ranging from the complexities of conceptualization to the thorny problems of data collection.[4] Yet the simple fact is that meaningful urban analysis and decision-making are next to impossible without "accounting for" a region's stocks or assets.

1. PROBLEMS OF GOVERNMENT DECISION-MAKING

When the design of a system of regional accounts is considered, the information requirements of public decision-making in urban regions deserve particular attention. These areas, which include the great bulk of the nation's population, require enormous investments in capital overhead, as well as complicated and expensive public services, in order to survive as efficient places for production and as desirable environments for family living. The needs to be met are great and the resources available limited, so that even under the most favorable political and economic conditions the problem of making choices is a difficult one.

There are several major focuses of governmental decision-making in urban communities. These are: (1) the provision of public services, including both personal services (health, education, welfare, etc.) and services for property (such as fire protection); (2) the

---

ships refer to the induced effect on capital formation of an increased demand for the region's output. These would be analogous to accelerator coefficients, with "capital formation" broadly conceived.

[4] See National Bureau of Economic Research, *Output, Input and Productivity Measurement*, Vol. 25 of Studies in Income and Wealth (Princeton: Princeton University Press, 1961).

physical development of the region, including planning, zoning, transportation, and renewal; (3) the economic development of the region, involving a concern for jobs and income; and (4) the financing of the governmental activities. Significantly, all of these are closely related, even if the relationships are not always recognized. Also, decisions have to be made with respect to the quantity and quality of particular stocks of assets as well as to the rate of flow of various current activities. Thus we need to develop an accounts model that will not only relate the various focuses of government decision-making but also incorporate both the stock and flow dimensions of these decisions.

Regional accounts can make a significant contribution to local decision-making precisely by organizing data so that they not only are helpful in decisions on specific subjects—say, an appropriate strategy for the development of the downtown area—but can bring key relationships to the forefront—for example, by indicating the probable effects of a given type of physical development on property values and the community's tax receipts. In other words, it is not enough to see to it that a large amount of helpful data are readily available; critical features of urban development must be sharply and usefully highlighted. Regional accounts should be as revealing of the main factors in urban development as national accounts are of the key factors in cyclical ups and downs. Brief reference to some of the key relationships will serve to illustrate the informational requirements in urban decision-making.

Governmental services and developmental efforts in urban communities are mainly directed at *people* and *property*. The quantity and characteristics of the population and the property determine in very large part what the government is called on to do and its ability to finance the required activities. These, in turn, are mainly functions of the economic structure of the urban region and particularly the kinds of industries it contains. The rate of growth (or decline) of such industries, their capital-labor ratios, and the levels of wages and profits will determine the jobs and income available in the community. Jobs and income, in turn, will tend to determine the total population of the community and its characteristics (age, sex, income level, occupation type, to some extent race, and the like) as well as the kinds of property which it will contain. A modifying factor will be the attraction of the community for retired and other non-job-oriented persons. However, in most communities such persons are a relatively small proportion of the total. And all this brings us back to the first point; namely, that the quantity and characteristics of the people and property will have a great deal to do with the kinds of services that the government will have to provide as well as the region's ability to pay for them.

To take only one example—a relatively uncomplicated one—of the kind of decision-making problems common in urban communities, we might refer to the question of school construction. It is apparent that if adequate school capacity is to be available within a given community, there will need to be information on a number of subjects, including existing school capacity and its use, anticipated school population and its characteristics, and school construction costs (for alternative size units, including costs of moving children in the case of larger units), as well as other anticipated demands for public expenditures and the total financial resources that can be counted on. The route to an estimate of future school population is by way of projected total population, based on projected job levels.

The linkages are, of course, much more complex in the case of public efforts toward physical and economic development. But here, just as much as in public services, numbers and characteristics of persons and property are key factors, so that estimation of jobs and income is critically important. This fact, in turn, underlines the central role of analysis of regional "comparative advantage" in order to get a usable fix on anticipated regional growth and change. A core problem is to evaluate what is happening to the economy of a given region, in relation to other regions, and what is likely to happen in the face of anticipated national growth and change.[5]

The main point is that if regional accounts are to be really helpful in decision-making they must be revealing of the key features of urban development, making possible—with the application of other tools—useful projections, impact analysis (i.e., the analysis

---

[5] This subject is discussed in the Perloff, Borts-Stein, and Delwart-Sonenblum papers in Hochwald, *op. cit.*

of alternative policies and expenditures), and a deeper understanding of urban change.[6]

2. A NOTE ON THE NATURE OF VARIOUS KINDS OF ACCOUNTS AND THEIR USES

An important limitation in the development of regional accounts at this stage is the fact that we do not have a fully articulated and empirically substantiated theory of regional growth. What we do have is a partial theory, which can be employed as a central organizing principle in the evolution of an accounts framework.[7] With an enrichment of the accounts data—providing directly comparable information for different regions and at different points in time—it should become possible to test out various suggestive hypotheses and compress the time needed for empirical establishment of a rounded theory of regional development.

The development of regional accounts is much influenced by the progress which has been made in social-accounts analysis in general. The theory and methods of regional accounts have evolved to a considerable extent out of the earlier traditions of national accounts, in particular the United States income and product and interindustry accounts. In many respects this development has been advantageous. Frequently theoretical notions, methodological conceptions, and empirical techniques found in the general literature on social accounts have been useful directly, or with minor modification, in the development of regional accounts. But this evolutionary development has had disadvantages too. In particular, it has tended to impose a preconceived pattern of functional concept and analytical relevance on the methodology of regional accounts.

There are, clearly, important distinctions between regional and

---

[6] Werner Hirsch has made a number of extremely valuable proposals for impact analysis in his paper in *Design of Regional Accounts* and in other papers, particularly his "Three Studies in the Measurement of the Impact of Metropolitan Growth" (Washington: Resources for the Future, Inc., mimeo, 1959).

[7] See items cited in footnote 5; also Barbara R. Berman, Benjamin Chinitz, Edgar M. Hoover, *Projection of a Metropolis* (Cambridge: Harvard University Press, 1961).

national accounts, particularly in that the analytical objectives with respect to which regional accounts typically are formulated, at least implicitly in terms of the problems which they are expected to illuminate, are generally different from those of national accounts. At the present time, the national accounts are used primarily to analyze questions of short-run cyclical stability, while regional accounts typically are employed in the analysis of long-run secular trends or structural change. For example, the national income and product accounts are used mainly as a framework for short-run projections of income, product, and employment in the context of a fixed labor supply, fixed natural resources, a capital supply which, if variable, varies in some known or knowable way, and, in addition, a fixed technology, i.e., ordinarily no account is taken of possible shifts in marginal productivity schedules for any factors of production.[8] Similarly, conventional interindustry analysis is focused on the effect on specific activity levels of changes in the final bill of goods, given a fixed technology, either fixed capacities or capacities subject to change only according to some fixed rules, and a constrained supply of at least some basic inputs. Whether or not they reflect the absence of secular growth as an important national goal prior to the very recent past, it is clear that the kinds of social accounts that have been constructed at the national level are not fully appropriate for describing past growth in analytically meaningful terms, much less for providing insight into what might be done to enhance future growth at a capacity level of operation of the system as a whole.

The analysis of secular change directly involves the consideration of changes in precisely those elements that are usually regarded as fixed in the analysis of cyclical stability and, in addition, of the interaction of such structural changes with the pattern of economic flows itself. In short, a broader range of phenomena than those traditionally treated must be considered within the accounts themselves if regional accounts are to be effective in the analysis of what

---

[8] This is not to say that national and regional accounts *could not* be used in the same way; it is simply to say that they *are not*. And this has important implications for the way the data are collected and organized.

appear to be the most pressing problems for regional, and particularly urban, economies.

A system which can provide an information base for the recording and analysis of regional economic growth, as suggested above, would have to account for both the magnitude of economic flows and changes in stocks of reproducible resources over time. Basically, what is needed is a system which not only can record historical changes in the quantity and quality of resources but also can provide an analytical description of the relationships between changes in economic flows and subsequent changes in resource stocks and, in addition, the relationships between changes in stocks and subsequent changes in the levels and composition of flows. This suggests that three types of resources information are needed. Specifically, the accounts would have to include (1) an asset inventory, (2) the material for an analysis of flow-stock relationships, and (3) the material for an analysis of stock-flow relationships.[9]

It should be noted that a set of accounts for a single year, no matter how comprehensive, could not in principle serve the needs of the second two objectives. Because the accounts would represent an empirical implementation of a theory dealing with the relationships between current flows and changes in stocks over time, observations over time would be necessary for any hypothesis testing. Moreover, both because the observed stock-flow relationships for any particular year could not be regarded necessarily as equilibrium values and because the equilibrium adjustment to structural (i.e., developmental) change inevitably involves at least several years, comprehensive data on stocks and flows would have to be collected over a number of years in order to provide understanding of the process of regional economic development and a base of information for decision-making.

It will be noted that the recording of flow-stock and especially stock-flow relationships which the suggested accounts are designed

[9] A complete inventory might not be needed. To the extent that the productivity analysis to be discussed below could be framed in terms *only* of equations with only differences in stocks as independent variables, then an accurate system for reporting changes in, not total amounts of, stocks would suffice.

to encompass is to some extent simply another way of handling marginal-productivity analysis.[10] One might, then, raise the question why these kinds of relationships cannot be determined by microeconomic analysis. First of all, it should be noted that there is nothing in the social-accounts framework suggested below which is inconsistent with microanalytic investigation; in fact, the accounts data should make possible much more extensive microanalysis, the results of which it is to be expected would influence the accounts structure. However, since the process of understanding a regional economy involves more than the understanding of the response patterns of the individual decision-making units comprising it (in particular, the interaction between these units), it is necessary to design a framework which allows for determining the effects of changes in the flow from one unit on the flows emanating from all other units. And accounts models are designed precisely to focus on this kind of interaction.

From the foregoing it also should be clear that accounts models should be regarded in no sense as inconsistent or methodologically competitive with quantitative behavioral (i.e., econometric) models; quite the contrary: they are necessarily complementary. For example, accounts models, *by themselves*, are incapable of predicting anything at all about the future, at least so long as they contain independent variables (although they still would be useful in comparing the effects of alternative hypothetical changes in the independent elements of the system). On the other hand, while econometric models offer a means of predicting the future values of the independent variables, *by themselves* they provide no basis for deriving policy decisions from the predictions they supply. In short, if we have no basis for predicting an economy's final bill of goods, for example, a set of interindustry accounts is of limited significance in determining a region's future economic situation. On the other hand, without some kind of accounts model we have no basis for assessing the effects on the economy of predicted changes in the final bill of goods. In other words, in bridging the gap between

[10] Stating this relationship in terms of marginal productivity assumes, of course, that the basic accounts are disaggregated to a level of industrial detail sufficient to insure a reasonable degree of homogeneity within any given industrial class.

regional accounts and regional development policy we need to predict and we need to be able to analyze the significance of predicted changes, so that both accounts and econometric models must be brought into play in any analytical system designed to accommodate policy decision-making.[11]

The special requirements of regional analysis suggest that if the critical relationships as they evolve over time are to be kept front and center, regional accounts cannot necessarily limit themselves severely to reconcilable, transactor-based data. While such data must certainly make up the core of any accounts system, they can achieve their maximum usefulness only if they can be tied directly to *associated accounts* and other key *associated data* and into an integrated system which can more closely approximate a general equilibrium model. Unfortunately, we cannot yet, as discussed later, integrate all the key factors at once.[12] In the model discussed here the main focus is on the integration of key resource stocks within the accounts framework, but even these are necessarily limited. Thus, we cover only those resources which at the present time are amenable to measurement and to policy control, and with respect to which meaningful functional hypotheses seem likely to be made within our present knowledge.

3. RESOURCES AND FLOWS TO BE CONSIDERED

When we want to get at the fundamentals of regional growth, we find ourselves at once concerned with the key resources at the base

---

[11] Also either some concept of an objective function which the community hopes to maximize or a set of simulated results of policy alternatives must be provided. Moreover, even in the case of a simulation model some screening of both the criterion variables and the range of alternatives simulated must be made, and presumably on the basis of community preferences. The substantive problems in the evaluation of community goals will not, however, be considered here.

[12] For example, the authors have explicitly eliminated intersectoral money-flows data. Subsequent comments by Ruth P. Mack have suggested that this decision might be reconsidered. While earlier investigations tended to indicate that the intersectoral flows *internal* to the region may have little significance for regional capital formation, Dr. Mack has suggested that such flows may be significant in explaining other aspects of regional economic performance, in particular interregional price differentials.

of economic development; namely, human resources, natural resources, and capital resources (both private property and public social-overhead facilities). We want to work toward establishing relationships between changes in such resource stocks—either independent changes or changes induced by prior changes in flows—and subsequent changes in flows (i.e., in output, income, and employment).

Accounting for human-capital resources involves extremely difficult, but not insurmountable, problems. Thus, for example, where earlier it seemed impossible to conceive of a "value" figure for "human assets," the work on a lifetime-income measure suggests that such a measure can be both feasible and meaningful.[13] Unfortunately, we do not as yet have anything comparable in the field of natural resources.[14] The authors are well aware of the problems arising out of the tendency for the value of resource stocks to be largely demand-determined. For this reason we try to provide for the measurement of stocks in physical rather than value terms, where feasible.

If the economic flows prevailing at the time the accounts estimation begins can be regarded as approximating equilibrium levels, with respect to the then-existing resource stocks a rather substantial simplification can be achieved. If a start is made from equilibrium all subsequent changes in observed flows can be imputed to intervening changes in stocks (or a change in technology). But non-reproducible assets cannot have changed; hence the asset accounts in the system can be confined to reproducible assets. This restriction also assumes that the marginal productivity of non-reproducible assets is not affected by changes in the stock of reproducible resources. In the case of a region initially undeveloped such a limitation would be preposterous. But in the context of an established urban region it may not be serious. Even in achieving long-run equilibrium over a decade or so the probable change in the scale of activity is not likely to exceed 20 or 30 per cent. Also, the natural-resource component of inputs (other than land) in an urban region

[13] Burton A. Weisbrod, "An Expected-Income Measure of Economic Welfare," *Journal of Political Economy*, 70 (Aug. 1962), 355–67.
[14] Even here, though, step-by-step progress, as in the measurement of water availability, can one day provide an adequate basis for asset evaluation.

is likely to be small. Accepting these restrictions still leaves an extremely broad resource inventory, including not only structures but capital equipment and human resources, as well as land. Since the accounts are intended to cover relationships between reproducible resources and their space requirement, land itself (even though it is non-reproducible) would have to be included—and, fortunately, can be.

The question of land, and space requirements in general, is extremely important in regional analysis. Land use and land-use planning are at the center of many of the decisions made by both public and private units in the urban community. Both productive efficiency and family livability are directly related to space requirements. The space needs of business units, of public facilities, of homes, and of transportation [15] and recreation all have to be known and projected if appropriate provisions are to be made and physical development is to be properly channeled.[16]

Such space requirements and their "feedback" on the economic functioning of the region must be provided for in the accounts framework. Except those for transportation, however, most space requirements can be related directly to human and non-human resources. Thus, another contribution of an expanded accounts system may be to permit a more effective analysis of linkages between urban economic function and the pattern of land use by the relating of use requirements not to processes but directly to the resources which must be spatially accommodated.

On the flow side the problem of focus does not seem so severe; we already have some experience behind us. Essentially we want the accounts to include the measurement of those flows which indicate the nature of the region's economic structure and state of economic well-being at a given point in time, in a form which can

---

[15] Large amounts of space (in some cases as much as 40% of total land in cities) tend to be taken up by the requirements of vehicles for movement and parking.

[16] This suggests another criterion for delimiting the set of resources which should be included in the accounts: that they specifically require spatial accommodations, e.g., a locational designation or assignment. Data would be needed on the numbers of each kind of structure, including public buildings and residences, the density of travel between every pair of structures, and the amount of land required for recreational use.

permit meaningful analysis over time. While many troublesome problems remain here, there would seem to be widespread agreement on the use of output, income, and employment as the critical variables to be recorded and explained.[17]

4. AN INTEGRATED RESOURCES-FLOW ACCOUNT

We conceive of the *core account* within an expanded accounts system as covering the production and income data, and the *associated accounts* as covering the human resources and non-human resources designated earlier as holding a key place in regional analysis, and covering as well a government expenditure and revenue account. We conceive further that all the accounts would provide data on totals not only for the entire urban region but for designated districts within the region as well.

On the last point, it is obvious that the metropolitan area is anything but a "uniform plain." The downtown areas are very different from the suburbs, and each of these is made up of many types of communities, usually undergoing important changes of one kind or another. Many of the major urban decisions that are made concern developmental matters such as urban renewal and transportation or health and welfare considerations that must be given a specific locational assignment within the region. Decisions regarding such matters can be made sensibly only if there is a good bit of information available about the different communities and neighborhoods of the metropolis.

[17] Two possible criticisms which could be made concerning the use of these measures are that no account is taken either of price movements or of the distribution of income. Aside from the more extensive data requirements, there would seem to be no special problem in developing constant-dollar deflators for regions (as opposed to the nation). So far as the size distribution of income is concerned, substantial regional variation does exist and changes over time do occur even in individual regions. To the extent that this is true, such data could be developed independently of the accounts themselves. Leaving it out of the accounts essentially assumes away any relationship between the size distribution of income and either consumption or labor-force participation, given the rate of employment, average income, and the functional (or industrial) distribution of income, all of which would be included. This would seem a relatively modest concession in light of the probable cost of accounting for changes in size distribution on a current basis.

The basic form of a suggested schema which it is hoped will fulfill many of the foregoing objectives is outlined below. At this stage, it seems appropriate and probably possible only to set down a barebones description of the substance of the variables. Fuller development of the specifications of the system will probably have to await at least a preliminary attempt at an empirical implementation of the system outlined below or of one analogous to it.

5. CURRENT PRODUCTION AND INCOME ACCOUNT

The schematic designation of the Current Production and Income Account as shown in Figure 1 is intended to represent the set

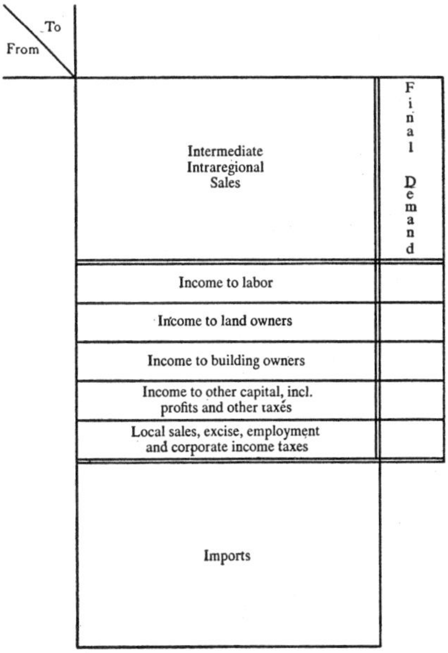

From \ To		
Intermediate Intraregional Sales		Final Demand
	Income to labor	
	Income to land owners	
	Income to building owners	
	Income to other capital, incl. profits and other taxes	
	Local sales, excise, employment and corporate income taxes	
Imports		

Figure 1. Current Production and Income Account

of integrated income-and-product-interindustry accounts developed earlier (only the summary account is shown, however; accounts for individual sectors of current activity are omitted).[18] In terms of account identities it could be written as follows:

[18] See Charles L. Leven, "Regional Income and Product Accounts: Construction and Applications," in Hochwald, *op. cit.*, pp. 148–95.

188 Toward an Integrated System of Regional Accounts

(1) $$X_1 = \sum_{j=1}^{n} t_{ij} X_j + Y_i \qquad (i=1, \ldots n)$$

(2) $$X_j = \sum_{i=1}^{n} (t_{ij} + m_{ij}) X_i + a_{Lj} \sum_{j=1}^{n} X_{Lj} + a_{Rj} \sum_{j=1}^{n} X_{Rj}$$
$$+ a_{Bj} \sum_{j=1}^{n} X_{Bj} + a_{Kj} \sum_{j=1}^{n} X_{Kj} + a_{sj} \sum_{c=1}^{n} R_{sj}$$
$$(j=1, \ldots n)$$

where

(3) $$t_{ij} = \frac{T_{ij}}{X_j}, \; m_{ij} = \frac{M_{ij}}{X_j} \text{ and } t_{ij} + m_{ij} = a_{ij} \qquad \begin{matrix}(i=1, \ldots n)\\(j=1, \ldots n)\end{matrix}$$

and

(4) $$\sum_{j=1}^{n} X_{Lj} + \sum_{j=1}^{n} X_{Rj} + \sum_{j=1}^{n} X_{Bj} + \sum_{j=1}^{n} X_{Kj} + \sum_{j=1}^{n} R_{Sj} + X_{LY} + X_{RY}$$
$$+ X_{BY} + X_{KY} = Y_p$$

where

(5) $$Y_R = Y_P = (T_{xz} - T_{zx})$$

where

$X_i =$ output of industry i
$Y_i =$ final demand for industry i
$T_{ij} =$ sales from industry i in the region to industry j in the region
$M_{ij} =$ imports of input i by industry j
$X_{Lj} =$ income to labor from industry j
$X_{Rj} =$ income to land owners from industry j
$X_{Bj} =$ income to building owners from industry j
$X_{Kj} =$ income to other capital, including profits and other taxes, from industry j
$R_{Sj} =$ local sales, excise, employment, and corporate income taxes paid by industry j
$a_{ij} =$ amount of input i needed per unit output of industry j $(i=1, \ldots n, L, R, B, K, S)$
$Y_p =$ income produced in the region
$Y_R =$ income received in the region
$T_{xz} =$ income, taxes, and other transfers out of the region
$T_{zx} =$ income and other transfers into the region.

As in the earlier accounts, governmental activity would be included in the interindustry-transaction matrix. User-cost-financed activities of local government (transit, power, etc.) could be treated as private producers, with any resulting surplus or deficit showing up in the profits row (within the cell corresponding to the column for the particular activity). Other activities of local government would be aggregated in a separate row (s) at the bottom, but *within* the interindustry section of the account, i.e., within the X_j.[19]

Those activities of state and federal government which were determined by the level of demand or activity in the region (highway maintenance or meat inspection) could be treated as quasi-private production, i.e., recorded in a separate row (s) in the matrix, with total output defined as being equal to purchases of goods and services with zero profits. The rest of state and federal activity would be put in the export component of the final-demand sector (i.e., treated as if it were physically removed from the area) or, in the case of a large region, prorated between in-region production and final demand.

A change from the conventions used in earlier interindustry analyses would be made in the case of rental-housing services, which would be defined as including the imputed rental value of owner-occupied housing. Also, both imputed and real output of residential housing rather than being assigned to final demand would be classed as an input to the industry or industries of employment of the regularly employed members of the household, with a corresponding subtraction from labor or proprietary earnings in those industries. In households not having any employed member, rental service would go directly to final demand. This adjustment would make possible a direct linkage between activity levels, by industry, and the stock of residential housing.

Somewhat special conventions would be employed in the case of taxation. State and federal sales and excise taxes would be netted

---

[19] In the case of government activities not technologically linked to any industrial process, but going *entirely* to final demand (a free zoo might be an example), there would be a technical problem of maintaining the non-singularity of the interindustry-transactions matrix because of the zero vector in the row for that activity within the matrix. Here the factor inputs could simply be rerouted directly into either the consumption vector or a special vector in final demand.

out of the system entirely and direct taxes of the state and federal governments would show up in the reconciliation between income produced in and that received by the region (as part of T_{xz} in equation 5). An exception would occur where state and federal activities were assigned or prorated to the regional-activity matrix. Then the amount of *all* state and federal taxes corresponding to the "output" of such activities would be assigned instead to the "local tax" row, R_{Sj}. In addition the R_{Sj} now would include taxes on regional production *activities*, which would thus be treated as inputs. These would include local sales, excise, employment, and corporation-income taxes. Local taxes on income and resources (i.e., poll, property, and personal-income taxes, estate taxes, and licenses) would be netted out of the private-activity rows and columns. In total they would show up as a positive input in the regional-government column in the "income to other capital, including profits and other taxes" row, X_{Kj}.

Final demand is shown as a single column, Y_i, simply for convenience in schematic representation. Actually several sectors of final demand would be employed (exports, local consumption, etc.) and individual sectors of current flow articulated.[20] The sum of the final-demand column, including the items in the factor-input rows, would represent gross product or income produced currently in the region. It would differ from the usual definition in that it would exclude sales and excise taxes paid to the state and federal governments. All other taxes would be included in the "local tax" row or residually in the row for "Income to other capital, including profits and other taxes."

Finally, it should be noted that the interindustry transactions are not exactly in the form of a standard input-output table. The upper matrix records only those interindustry transactions internal to the region; it is what has been designated a "from-to" table.[21] However, since the industrial breakdown of each industry's imports is shown in the lower matrix, the reconciliation between the "from-to" and "input-output" coefficients consists simply of adding the two matrices

---

[20] For a discussion of the problems of sectoring final demand, see Charles M. Tiebout, *Markets for California Products* (Sacramento: California Development Agency, 1961).

[21] See Charles L. Leven, in Hochwald, *op. cit.*

after they are normalized (this is indicated in equation 3). This is an alternative to the procedure used in the 1947 U.S. interindustry analysis, which shows imports of any given commodity as an import of the domestic producing industry and then as an intermediate transaction between that industry and the consuming one.[22] The reason for adopting the present convention is that where limitation of research resources requires, or similarity of regional and national technology permits, such a simplification, the import matrix can be compressed to a single row and determined as a residual. Earlier there was a reference to determining the "Income to other capital, etc." row as a residual. It would be possible to determine imports as a residual component of sales and still to determine income to other capital, etc., as a residual component of value added where an estimate of value added by industry independent of factor payments was available, i.e., a blow-up of "value added per employee" by the number of employees.

6. NON-HUMAN RESOURCES ACCOUNT

The Non-human Resources Account, shown in Figure 2, is simply a recording of the relevant non-human resources classified according to industry or activity (such as housing). To preserve a properly testable relationship between current flows and non-human resource stocks (equation 23) only the resources currently being used should be related to each current activity.

Thus, in the functional representation of the account below a distribution is made between total, utilized, and idle non-human resources.

(6) $$L = \sum_{i=1}^{n} L_i + L_o$$

(7) $$B = \sum_{i=1}^{n} B_i + B_o$$

(8) $$K = \sum_{i=1}^{n} K_i + K_o$$

[22] See W. Duane Evans and Marvin Hoffenberg, "The Interindustry Relations Study for 1947," *Review of Economics and Statistics*, 34 (May 1952), 97–142.

where

L_i = land area in industry i
B_i = building floor space in industry i
K_i = value of equipment in industry i
L_o = vacant land area
B_o = vacant floor space
K_o = idle equipment.

Also note that the account identities and the table (Figure 2) indicate an accounting for each of the three classes of non-human resources in a single dimension. This will be discussed below.

As far as totally idle resources are concerned, there seems to be no special accounting problem, except adjusting for resources totally idle during only part of the accounting period. Underemployed resources present more of a problem. The assumption that equilibrium values would be approximated by moving averages is not satisfactory in that the distribution of under- and over-capacity utilization is downward biased. A more favorable solution might be to estimate excess capacity by extrapolation between successive peaks in output over time.

In testing stock-flow relationships (e.g., equation 26), however, it would be necessary to have total resource stocks whether currently used or not. Thus the account includes a provision for accounting for vacant or idle resources. Depending on the detail employed in testing a relationship like equation 26, it might be necessary to have an industrial distribution of the vacant or idle row.

It might also be pointed out that certain problems might arise out of the degree of aggregation of individual activities used in the Current Production and Income Account. Specifically, the resource stocks of the government would be aggregated into only as many component activities as were individually designated in the production account. For example, aggregates like "street and highway transportation" and "public education" might be satisfactory for relating governmental activity to the industrial composition of current outputs. However, where significant and identifiable intra-activity variation in capital-output ratios existed, further disaggregation might be called for. The same might also be the case for private activities, especially housing services.

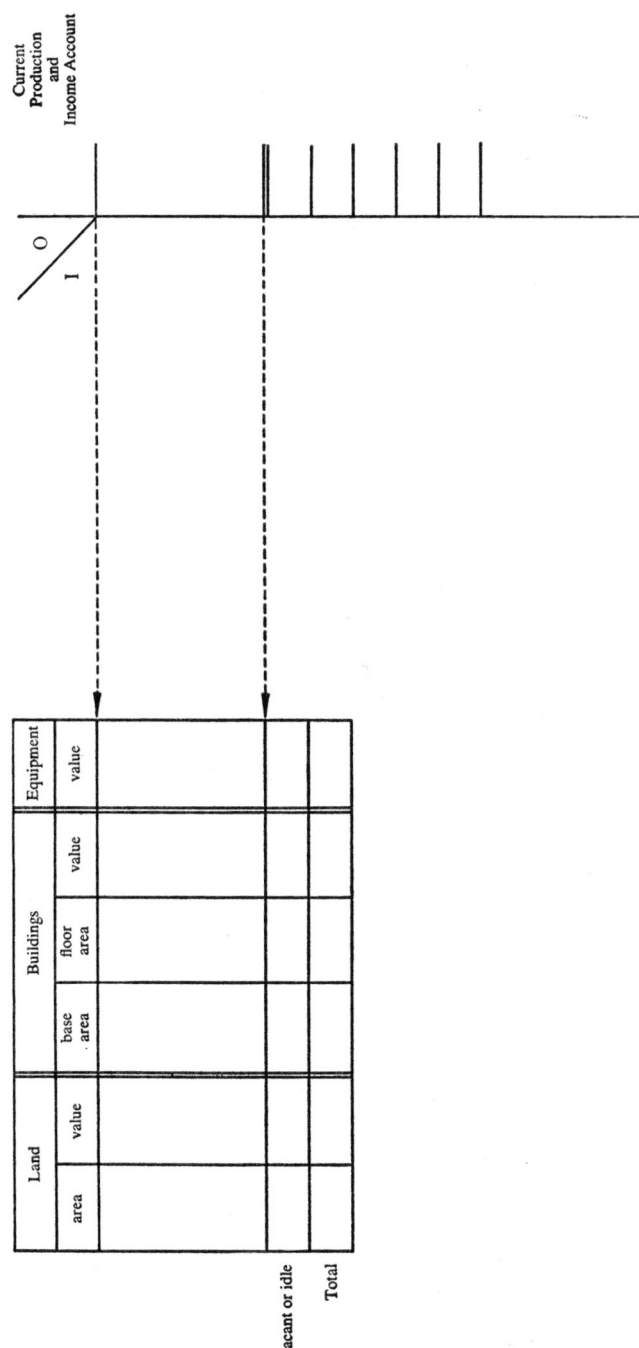

Figure 2. Non-human Resources Account

Another problem arises in specifying the amount of detail needed in the resource description for any given activity. It is clear that purely qualitative differences in resources of a given kind, say different kinds of capital equipment having the same monetary value, do produce differences in marginal productivity. However, our knowledge of such relationships is very limited. Also, to some extent they are eliminated by the market mechanism. For these reasons it would seem wise to introduce a conservative bias with respect to the proliferation of detailed qualitative resource description, at least at the present time. This is not to preclude the collection of such qualitative information subsidiary to the accounts.

At a minimum, simply the quantity of land might be recorded. The account, it will be noted, covers land value as well. However, since the price of land is so largely demand-determined, land value is included more as a variable to be explained (in particular, it is relevant to property-tax decisions) than as an explanatory one. In the case of buildings, both base and floor areas should be included to permit an analysis of the substitutability of height for base area. Also value can serve here as a proxy for quality. Finally, in the case of equipment the heterogeneity even within a single narrowly defined industry probably precludes anything more than a simple proxy. In this regard current market value seems preferable to depreciated original cost or replacement cost.

7. HUMAN RESOURCES ACCOUNT

The considerations involved in designing the Human Resources Account (Figure 3) are similar to those involved in non-human resources. The account includes both employment, E_i, for flow-stock analysis (equation 24) and labor force, W_i, for stock-flow analysis (equation 26). In addition, by the inclusion of both total and resident employment in each industry (the difference between these two figures would represent in-commuters [23]) as well as out-commuters, a reconciliation between total employment in the region and total employment of the region's residents can be achieved. In

[23] For convenience this distinction is not shown in the identities below.

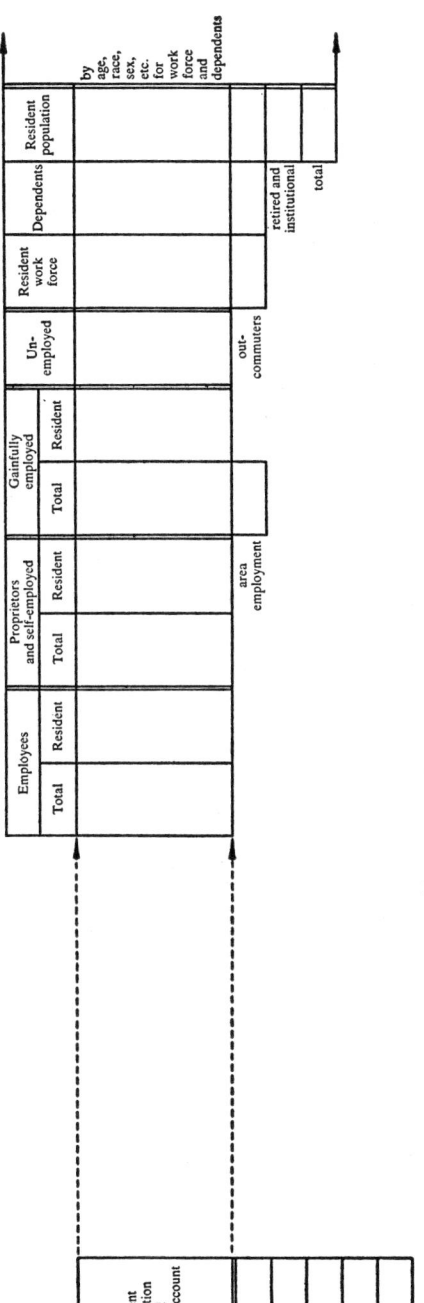

Figure 3. Human Resources Account

serving the needs of an analysis of labor-force productivity, an industrial distribution of out-commuters as well might be called for, but this is not shown in the identities below by industry, but only in the aggregate, W_c. The accounts (although again for convenience, not the identities) also distinguish between employees and proprietors and self-employed. This distinction is mainly a reflection of the asymmetric data sources in the two categories.

The Human Resources Account also includes the linkage between labor force and population, by recording the dependent population associated with each member of the labor force. Here it would seem reasonable to assign each working member to the industry of his employment and to assign other members of the household to the industry of employment of the primary worker. Finally, retired and institutional population would also be included to account for total population. Note that total population too is indicated functionally by a single variable, P. This is meant to stand for a good deal of socioeconomic detail as indicated in Figure 3. With the simplifications indicated the identities for this account would appear as follows:

(9) $$E = \sum_{i=1}^{n} E_i$$

(10) $$W_i = E_i + U_i \qquad (i = 1, \ldots n)$$

(11) $$W = \sum_{i=1}^{n} W_i + W_c$$

and

(12) $$P_i = W_i + D_i \qquad (i = 1, \ldots n)$$

and

(13) $$P = \sum_{i=1}^{n} P_i + W_c + D_c + P_r$$

where
- U_i = employment in industry i
- E_i = work force in industry i
- W_i = unemployed labor force last employed in industry i
- D_i = dependents of work force in industry i
- P_i = population associated with industry i
- W_c = out-commuting work force
- D_c = dependents of out-commuting work force

P_r = retired and institutional population
P = population.

As indicated earlier, the key assumption is that population is a dependent variable, except for retired and institutional population, P_r, and is a function of labor demand (see equations 24 and 25). Essentially, this assumes that in the long run workers move, at least at the margin, where economic opportunity arises. The proportion of retired and institutionalized people in the total population could be assumed to follow some determinable trend. For regions having special attraction to retired people or immigrants, especially from minority groups, independent estimates might have to be made.

Again, as in the case of non-human resources, decisions have to be made as to the degree of detail in the resource inventory. Here it would seem a much greater degree of detail is called for. First, we do know a good deal about the kinds of qualitative characteristics which affect labor productivity; for example, there is little doubt that at least age, sex, and level of education do make a difference. Second, there is less reason here to suppose that earnings differentials are a good proxy for productivity differentials than in the case of non-human resources. The market seems to be much more prone to discriminate against old people, women, or Negroes than against buildings and machinery which are either old or the "wrong" color. Some of the characteristics to be included have been noted above. We might also want other items too, like place of birth, years of residence in the region, and mortality and selected morbidity rates. Still greater detail is called for by the requirement to develop specific ties to the Regional Government Account. This point is discussed later. The precise breakdown has been indicated in the table simply as an "open end." A more precise determination of the optimum breakdown will have to rely on later study.

8. REGIONAL GOVERNMENT ACCOUNT

Certain key problems in analyzing local-government activity have been discussed earlier.[24] So far as the inclusion of product produced

[24] See Leven and Perloff papers in Hochwald, *op. cit.*

in the local government sector is concerned there is no real problem. If we are willing to stick with the convention that the value of government product is equal to its factor cost, then it is already included in the Current Production and Income Account.[25]

The real problem arises when an attempt is made to relate local-government expenditures and receipts to individual activity levels in the region. The most serious problem in this regard is on the expenditure side. Suppose we want to analyze the impact of changes in business activity on government-service (i.e., current-expenditure) requirements on the basis of the Current Income and Production Account alone. This account would indicate the average (or marginal, in the case of accounts over time) capacity of each industry to pay taxes, but this would be a very poor indicator of its capacity to consume most government services. True, an increase in activity in any given industry would add workers, hence population, hence school children, hence, the need for school expansion. But it is the increase in school children which has to be serviced, and the requirements are independent of the identity of the industry, given the size of the induced population increase, and certainly are independent of that industry's capacity to pay school taxes.

What we must do is trace through the relationships between the Current Production and Income Account and the Human Resources Account and then between the latter and the expenditure side of the Regional Government Account (Figure 4). Except for some services in support of transportation and certain recreational services (these would be included in "Other expenditures"), almost all local-government outlays would be related to the stock of resources, human and non-human, rather than to current activity levels. For example, fire protection is related to the number and kind of structures and the extent of land they occupy much more than to industrial output; police protection is related to the number of people more than to the number of man-hours worked. This fact requires the determination of the human and non-human resources in any

[25] And there would be no problem in determining gross product originating specifically in government since government activities would be carried in separately identifiable rows in the current account, i.e., where there were k separate government activities they would be represented by $X_{n-k}, \ldots, X_n$ in equation 1.

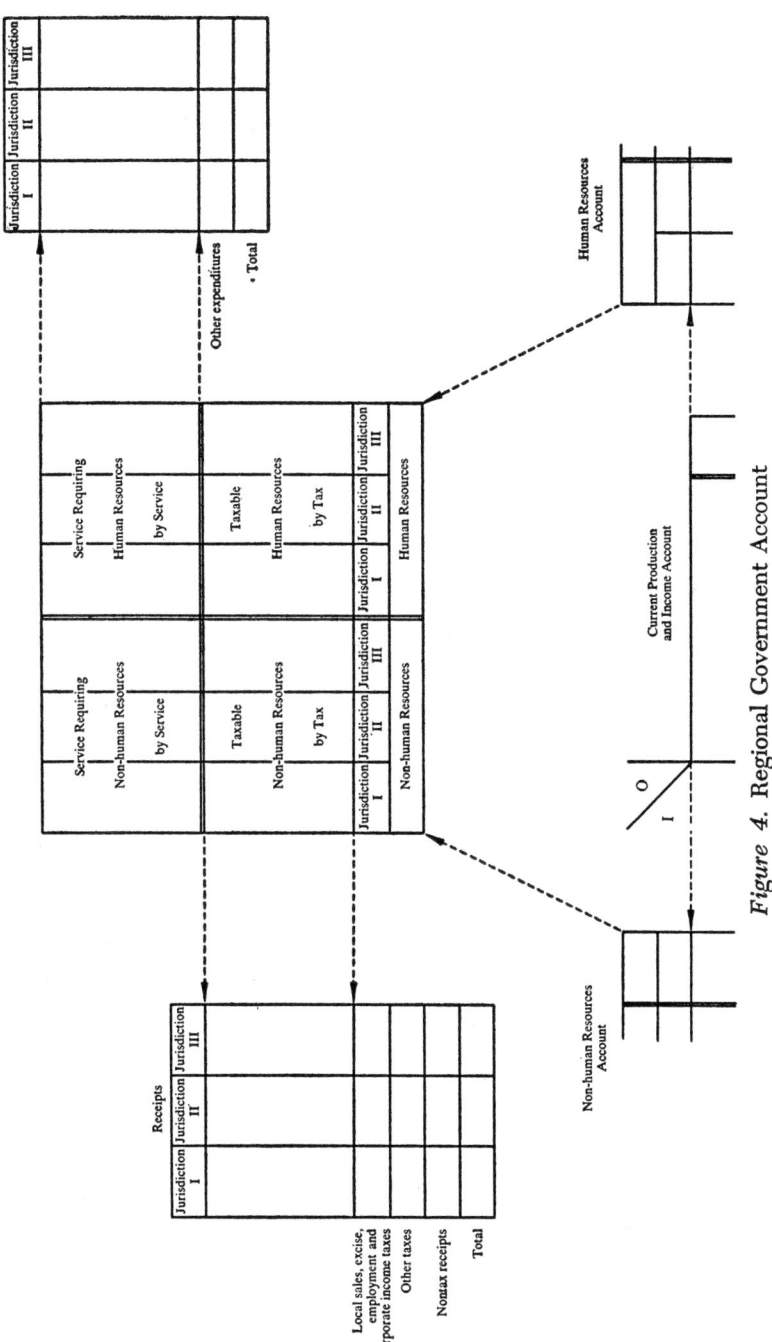

Figure 4. Regional Government Account

given local-government jurisdiction which consume *each kind* of public service provided by that jurisdiction.[26] Note that if this assignment could be made, the marginal propensity of each group to consume each service could be estimated by a set of accounts over time. Moreover, even in the absence of specific estimates of these propensities, the wealth of data on the relationship between human assets and government services would be a major contribution to the understanding of this difficult area.

What is particularly important for decision-making is the relationships between the need for public services, on one side, and the characteristics of the population of the metropolis and its sub-communities on the other. The elements to be "accounted for" are then: (a) the total population of the metropolis seen as recipients of each of the public services; and (b) the public services—specifically, the operating and capital expenditures for each service (education, health, police, housing, transportation, recreation, welfare, etc.).

Thus, for example, all persons attending public schools would be accounted for under the "education services" row in the top half of the right side of the central table in Figure 4. Each cell in the row would indicate the number of school children in the jurisdiction pertaining to that column. Adding across jurisdictions would give total school children in the region. Total education expenditures would be recorded in the corresponding row of the subsidiary table on the right.

Those receiving the service might be called the "subject" or "client" population. Figures would be provided for the *actual* subject population on a *full-time-equivalent* basis. This would show, for example, how many persons in each age group actually attended school last year measured in terms of full-time-equivalent units. The potential subject population might also be recorded (this would be based on a specified standard set by law, custom, or

[26] The resources using different services are not mutually exclusive, i.e., the columns would not add to the total population, or land, or buildings (this is indicated by equations 20 and 21). In fact, since most people would require several kinds of services, each half-column would add to much more than the total of the resource recorded in that half-column (the columns are divided in two, the top half covering services and the bottom half, receipts).

professional recommendation). In making projections the interplay between needs and/or demands on one hand and standards for the public service on the other would thus be brought to the fore and comparisons with "performance" in previous years and in other areas would be possible.[27]

Education expenditures, broken down by major categories (e.g., those for grade schools, high schools, colleges, technical schools), should be recorded for both operating and capital items (although this distinction is not indicated explicitly in the identities below or in Figure 4). This procedure would provide data, by extension, on a per-pupil basis and permit comparisons with the past and with other communities in this regard.

For most public services, the subject (or client) populations, both actual and potential, would differ; in a few cases the total population would be covered, as in certain of the general protective services. Thus, the notion of a "potential" subject population is useful not only in measuring performance but also in making projections of future requirements for public services. On the basis of these considerations, the identities for Figure 4 would appear as follows:

(14) $$\sum_{g=I}^{III} (L+B+K)^g \geq (L+B+K)$$

(15) $$\sum_{g=I}^{III} P^g \geq P$$

(16) $$R_r^g = q_r [(L+B+K)_r^g + P_r^g] \quad (r=1,\ldots R) \quad (g=I, II, III)$$

(17) $$N_n^g = v_n [(L+B+K)_n^g + P_n^g] \quad (n=1,\ldots N) \quad (g=I, II, III)$$

where

---

[27] The role of changing standards would also be recorded in this way. For example, the number of persons not attending school within each age group would be shown, as well as the number of drop-outs, and year by year the improvement or decline in educational performances could be shown (i.e., after the accounts had been kept for a number of years). Needless to say the authors recognize that quality of public services could be analyzed only to a very limited extent with the proposed tools. But since this issue is so important it would seem worth while to provide for whatever analysis of this type would be feasible with data available on a continuing basis.

(18) $$R^g = \sum_{r=1}^{R} (R_r^g + R_s^g + R_d^g + R_o^g) \qquad (g = I, II, III)$$

(19) $$N^g = \sum_{n=1}^{N} (N_n^g + N_o^g) \qquad (g = I, II, III)$$

but

(20) $$(L+B+K)^g \leq \sum_{r=1}^{R} (L+B+K)_r^g + \sum_{n=1}^{N} (L+B+K)_n^g \qquad (g = I, II, III)$$

(21) $$P^g \leq \sum_{r=1}^{R} P_r^g + \sum_{n=1}^{N} P_n^g \qquad (g = I, II, III)$$

where

$(L+B+K)^g$ = non-human resources in jurisdiction g
P^g = human resources in jurisdiction g
R^g = receipts in jurisdiction g
N^g = expenditures in jurisdiction g
$(L+B+K)_r^g$ = non-human resources in jurisdiction g subject to tax r
P_r^g = human resources in jurisdiction g subject to tax r
$(L+B+K)_n^g$ = non-human resources in jurisdiction g requiring expenditure n
P_n^g = human resources in jurisdiction g requiring expenditure n
R_r^g = receipts from tax r in jurisdiction g, for resource-related taxes
R_s^g = sales, excise, employment, and corporate-income-tax receipts in jurisdiction g
R_d^g = other tax receipts in jurisdiction g
R_o^g = non-tax receipts in jurisdiction g
N_o^g = non-resource-related expenditures in jurisdiction g

One of the main problems is to minimize the number of demographic characteristics employed, in order not to get bogged down in peripheral detail (and great expense). The characteristics which seem to be key to almost all public services are: age, sex, race, ethnic grouping, income, labor-force status, density, and residential stability (i.e., whether the population of the neighborhood or community is relatively stable or transient). However, the characteristics to be employed are, of course, analytical variables and additional study is needed to identify them specifically.[28] Note that allowance is made for the possibility of more than one governmental unit belonging to the region. Also, a particular resource might be in more than one jurisdiction so that the rows will not necessarily add to regional totals (see equations 14 and 15).

Finally, it should be noted that filling out the body of the Regional Government Account involves more than following the conventions implied by an accounting identity, as is the case in the rest of the accounts. In relationships 18 and 19, the jurisdictional distribution of resources is determinable by the application of jurisdictional definitions. But relationships 16 and 17 are true equations, not identities, and must be admitted to imply more than the usual kind of accounting procedure. Their validity, in fact, would have to be tested by the accounts data themselves. What this means is that initially this account might have to be based on some fairly clumsy *ad hoc* theorizing.

Things are a bit simpler on the receipts side. First, a number of taxes are linked directly to industrial activities, in particular sales, excise, employment, and corporation-income taxes. These would already have been adequately accounted for in the Current Production and Income Account and are carried simply as a summary item

---

[28] The usefulness of both the human resources and the government account could be enhanced if the data coverage were extended to all service provisions within the main service categories—including voluntary and private provision of services as well as public. If this were done, then private and parochial schools would be included under education services, and voluntary health and welfare expenditures would be shown as well as public health and welfare outlays. Not only would the picture be more complete, but the service expenditures could be totaled (given a residual "other services expenditures") and tied to the household items in the flow account. But this is the type of extension that is better left for later. One of the other extension possibilities is the tying in of data on the state of the physical facilities (the schools, hospitals, fire stations, etc.). It seems evident that to arrive at an estimate of capital requirements and future capital expenditures it is necessary to know about the state of the facilities and rate of depreciation and obsolescence. Even the roughest of estimates would be better than none, since it would alert the governmental authorities (and the public) to the future replacement situation. Whether it is feasible to make these estimates or not is another matter. Formally these data would appear in the government rows in the Non-human Resources Account.

in the "Receipts" table of this account. Moreover, at least the impact, if not the incidence, of the remaining major local-government taxes, real- and personal-property taxes, personal-income or wage taxes, and licenses is identifiable, i.e., equation 16 is much easier to approximate than 17.

9. INTRAREGIONAL ACCOUNT

As suggested earlier, the inclusion of the Intraregional Account in the system is a recognition of the importance of internal spatial arrangements in an urban complex. The account, as it stands here, involves nothing more than a recording of the location of employment, output, and all human and non-human resources in the system. It should be pointed out that no real attempt is being made here to design an ideal form for an intraregional account. The design of transportation models, for example, is an extremely complicated feature within the whole complex of urban analysis. However, within a general comprehensive framework for empirical analysis of metropolitan areas, as we are attempting to construct here, at least some indication of the role of intraregional accounts within the general framework must be provided. That is the intent of this section; it is not meant to supply the details of an intraregional account.

One decision which has to be made even at this level of generality has to do with the unit of observation which would be used in designating location. The possibilities range from ward and census tract down through enumeration district, block, and ultimately even street address. Since nothing more is involved than recording location and since location must be recorded for every item in the resource inventory, the authors would lean toward using the smallest unit possible, given the degree of aggregation in which the resource inventory itself is kept. Besides, smaller units can always be aggregated for analytical purposes with little difficulty.

As noted above, we are leaving to others the task of designing the specifics of this account. We simply want to make sure that our data system will generate the information needed for *intra-*

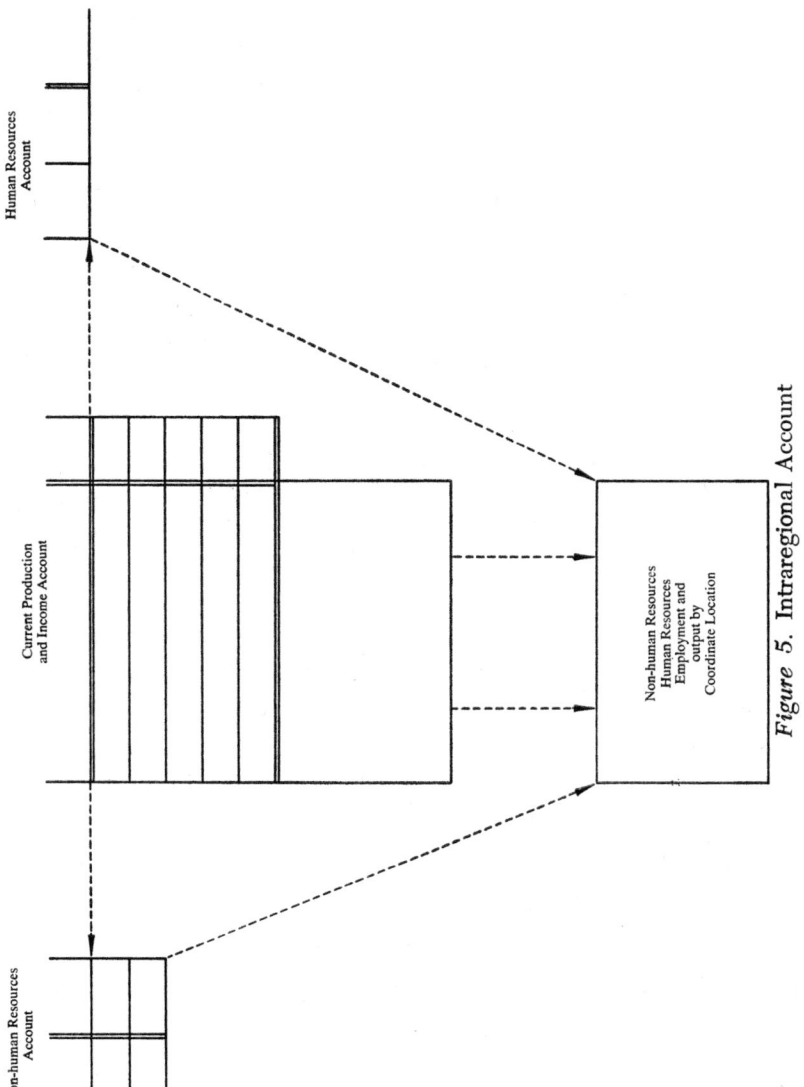

Figure 5. Intraregional Account

regional analysis. In this regard we are making one assumption, namely that the "transportation" problem and the "maximum productivity" problem can be solved, if not completely independently, at least iteratively. What this means is that we have a set of *regional* accounts (each for the region as a whole) [29] feeding into a single intraregional account.

The alternative would be to frame each of the four other accounts fully in terms of intraregional dimensions. This would internalize the whole question of intraregional adjustment within the general framework of analysis, rendering an intraregional account, per se, redundant. We have rejected this procedure on two counts. First, there seems to be some doubt at present as to our ability even to conceptualize the functional nature of a model of such generality in operationally observable terms. Second, given this doubt, one must take into account the vast increase in the cost of data collection that would be involved. In the present format, every piece of information in the other four accounts would have a regional "address" appended to it. This is the essence of what would be included in the Intraregional Account as indicated in Figure 5. The more general model, which we are rejecting, at least for the time being, would require, in addition to the "address" of each item, the specific spatial interchange between each item in any one of the accounts and, in general, each of the items in every other account as well. Within our concepts the Intraregional Account could be represented as:

$$(22) \qquad (L,B,K,P,E,X) = \sum_{m=1}^{M} \sum_{n=1}^{N} (L,B,K,P,E,X)_{mn}.$$

10. USING THE ACCOUNTS TO TEST RELATIONSHIPS

As indicated at the beginning, the major purpose of the accounts system herein proposed is to provide data organized in a form useful for testing hypotheses about regional economic and governmental

---

[29] In the Regional Government Account the geographic breakdown that would result would be only an incidental consequence of the jurisdictional breakdown.

functioning. The accounts system admittedly represents a considerable expansion in scope and complexity over those earlier employed, but an expansion which is essential if we are to enlarge our understanding of the urban-growth process. In short, if we are to meet this need we must press our information systems further.

But simply increasing the information flow is not enough. There are too many problems which conceivably could be investigated and almost limitless amounts of data which could be collected. The very magnitude of the task requires us to develop a sense of priority and a sense of proportion. We must be able to discriminate between vitally needed data and interesting information. It is hoped that this paper has made some contribution to that end. In this regard, the basic principle followed was to develop an accounts system which, if implemented over time, would permit the testing of relationships like these:

A. *Flow–Stock Equation (Non-human Resources)*

(23) $\qquad (L,B,K)_{i_{t+1}} = f_i(X_{i_t}) \qquad (i = 1, \ldots n)$

B. *Flow–Stock Equation (Human Resources)*

(24) $\qquad E_{i_{t+1}} = g_i(X_{i_t}) \qquad (i = 1, \ldots n)$

or, alternatively,

(24a) $\qquad (L,B,K,E)_{i_{t+1}} = L_i(X_{i_t}) \qquad (i = 1, \ldots n)$

and

(25) $\qquad D_{i_{t+1}} = k_i(W_{i_t}) \qquad (i = 1, \ldots n,c)$

C. *Stock–Tax Flow Equation*

(16) $\qquad R^g_{r_t} = q_r[(L+B+K)^g_r + P^g_r]_{t-1} \qquad \begin{array}{l}(r = 1, \ldots R)\\ (g = I, II, III)\end{array}$

D. Stock–Expenditure Flow Equation

(17) $\quad N^g_{n_t} = v_n[(L + B + K)^g_n + P^g_n]_{t-1} \quad \begin{array}{l}(n = 1, \ldots N) \\ (g = I, II, III)\end{array}$

E. Integrated Stock–Flow Equation

(26)

$$X^g_{i_t} = s_i(L_i + L_o, B_i + B_o, K_i + K_o, W_i, R^g, N^g)_{t-1} \quad \begin{array}{l}(i = 1, \ldots n) \\ (g = I, II, III)\end{array}$$

F. Intraregional Flow Equations

(27) $\quad X_{mn} = t_{mn}[(L,B,K,P,E,X)_{11}, \ldots, \quad (L,B,K,P,E,X)_{MN}] \\ \hphantom{(27) \quad X_{mn} = t_{mn}[(L,B,K,P,E,X)_{11}, \ldots,} \quad (m = 1, \ldots M) \\ \hphantom{(27) \quad X_{mn} = t_{mn}[(L,B,K,P,E,X)_{11}, \ldots,} \quad (n = 1, \ldots N)$

and

(28) $\quad T_{m-m', n-n'} = u_{mn}[(P,E,X)_{11}, \ldots, \quad (P,E,X)_{MN}] \\ \hphantom{(28) \quad T_{m-m', n-n'} = u_{mn}[(P,E,X)_{11}, \ldots,} \quad (m = 1, \ldots M) \\ \hphantom{(28) \quad T_{m-m', n-n'} = u_{mn}[(P,E,X)_{11}, \ldots,} \quad (n = 1, \ldots N)$

where

X_{mn} = output at location m,n.
$T_{m-m', n-n'}$ = transportation between m,n and m',n'.

Admittedly, as indicated above, these equations are not all that might be hoped for. They are no more than general expressions of what we are looking for. A detailed specification of their form probably must await the completion of some accounts-data collection and some preliminary testing. Nevertheless, it seems important to indicate at this time the nature of the functional ties between the accounts, even if only somewhat generally. The role of these relationships to the accounts system is indicated by the circled letters in Figure 6, which summarizes the proposed accounts system. Each circled letter refers to the corresponding equations above. The positions of the major variables in the accounts also are indicated in the summary figure.

Finally, it should be noted that the equations above are listed

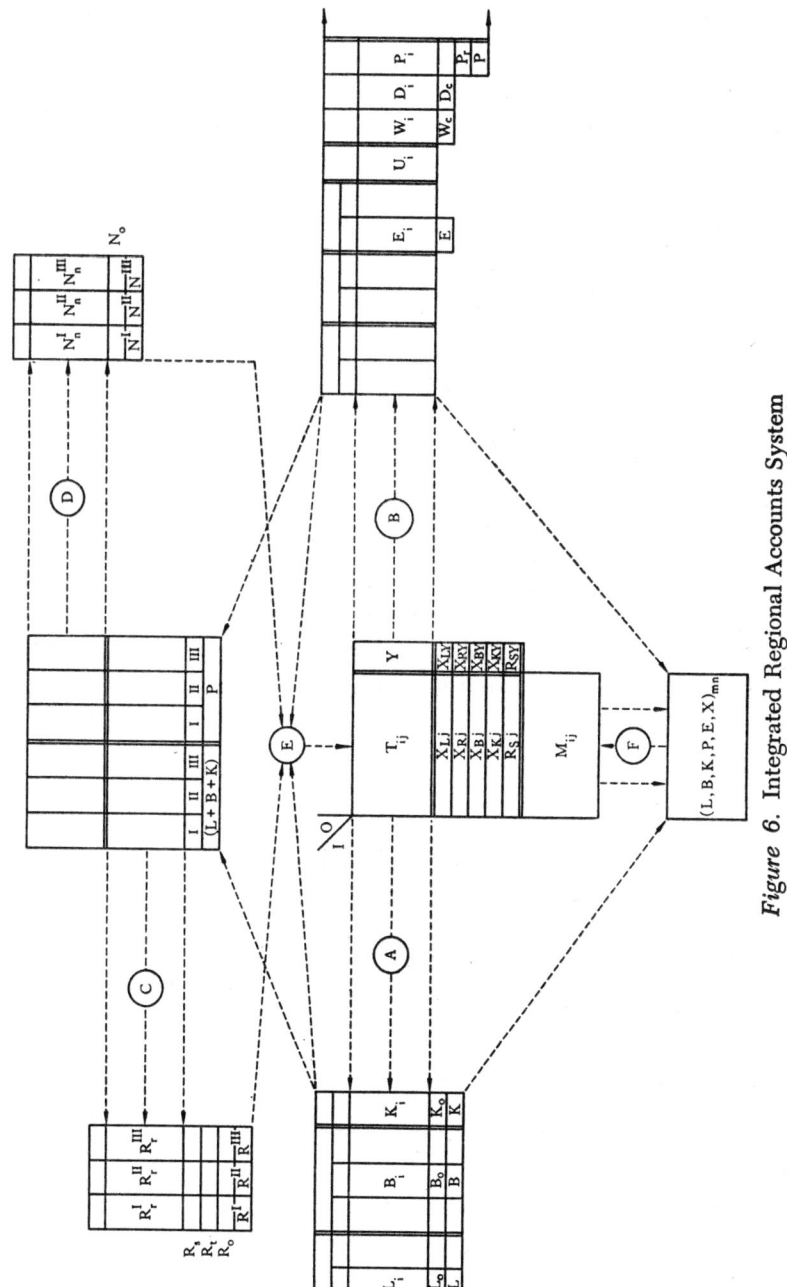

Figure 6. Integrated Regional Accounts System

more or less in order of their likely difficulty of implementation. At least the information for equations 23, 24, 24a, and 25 seems producible, perhaps with much effort but not too much conceptual difficulty. Equations 16 and 17 present the thorny problem of the connection between testing the relationships and generating the data for their testing, as indicated earlier.[30] While we have excused ourselves somewhat from the question of transportation models, we do recognize the great difficulties involved. Of the two general kinds of relationships which the Intraregional Account is designed to test, equations 26 and 27, the latter seems by far the more significant in terms of the prospect of obtaining useful results. It is intended to represent an urban transportation model.[31] Equation 26, the effect of the spatial pattern on productivity, is somewhat more doubtful of implementation. We would hope that further research might provide the necessary materials here. It is a subject that deserves attention, given the sweeping developmental decisions that need to be made in urban regions with regard to zoning, subdivision control, transportation, redevelopment, and related measures. This, of course, is only one of the many subjects touched on superficially in this paper which call for research in depth.

COMMENT

WERNER Z. HIRSCH
University of California, Los Angeles

Once again Leven and Perloff have given us an exciting and thought-provoking paper that deals with some of the more difficult aspects of regional accounts. It is indeed a pioneering venture and attempts to design an integrated system of flow and stock accounts

[30] See p. 203 above.
[31] For further details of such models, see Britton Harris paper, above.

within which key urban decision-making can be facilitated. Government decision-making focuses on the provision of public services, that is, on both operating and maintenance and investment decisions and the financing of the operating and capital budgets of government. These decisions should be planned so that they are consistent with the hopes and aspirations of the area's people, especially decisions involving employment and income.

The paper recognizes the important linkages between flow and stock, government and human resources, government and non-human resources, and human and non-human resources. It suggests an accounts framework within which these linkages are made explicit and can be studied. Few will disagree with the paper's assumption that the number of people and amount of property, and the characteristics of both, have much to do with the kinds of services that the government must provide. In brief, it assumes that government responds to needs but does not anticipate them, and while this is most likely realistic, some of us would favor more enterprise and leadership in government.

Recently René Dubos, in examining the question of whether man can keep up with history, pointed out that even the formulation of adequate goals for social development is far more difficult today than it was during earlier phases of civilization. His conclusion, no doubt correct, especially plagues the regional-accounts builder, who must digress in so many directions, many of them hardly reconcilable.

Therefore, it is all too understandable that Leven and Perloff compare different types of accounts. They conclude that there is an important distinction between regional and national accounts, in that the former are used mainly in the analysis of long-run secular trends or structural change, the latter in connection with short-run cyclical problems. But there are other differences, possibly no less important, which bear upon the design of the regional-accounts system. Other great issues are size and complexity of the rest-of-the-world sector, large-scale instability in the local structural coefficients, and the vagueness and yet complexity of local areas' goals.

Moreover, the authors suggest that "what is needed is a system which not only can record historical changes in the quantity and quality of resources," and as if that were not enough, they go on to say, "but also can provide an analytical description of the relationships between changes in economic flows and subsequent changes in resource stocks and, in addition, the relationships between changes in stocks and subsequent changes in the levels and composition of flows." I agree, and I also admire their wisdom and courage. Having tried my hand, to a minor extent, at studying quality measurements at one point of time, and having become aware of the enormous difficulties one encounters, I am overwhelmed by the suggestion of studying historical changes in quantity and quality. It is not only the quality of the asset that needs to be defined and ascertained but also the quality of that portion of the output that can be traced directly to the operating budget. In the case of public education, for example, this would mean measuring the quality not only of the capital assets but also of the rest of the school operation. I am most sympathetic to this point because I, too, have become convinced that in the urban-government sector, quality is a most important dimension. As a matter of fact, many of our local-government services cannot vary in quantity but merely in quality. Good examples are fire and police protection.

Turning now to a further aspect of the government account, I would like to applaud the useful distinction between those receipts that can be tied to business activity and those that cannot. Likewise, I agree with the conclusion that it is necessary to estimate the latter, as well as local-government expenditures outside the *core accounts*. While specific problems will call for different detail in the government-account breakdown, I would like to propose one facet that might fulfill many purposes. Specifically, I have in mind five major groupings: education and cultural services; protection, to include fire and police; roads, streets, and transportation; public health, welfare, and hospitals; and water, sanitation, and refuse collection. On the basis of the Leven-Perloff argument that user-cost-financed activities of local government could be treated as private producers, housing might be excluded from the public sector. This classification considers the extent to which the service fulfills social or merit wants and whether it is oriented toward human or non-human resources.

I would like to raise two further points briefly, although I am convinced that the authors are fully aware of them. The first is in the form of a question, namely, whether Figures 2 and 3, and to some extent Figure 4, are not asking for too much information. More specifically, I am wondering whether it would not be possible to spell out in more detail which bits of information are more essential than others. This is a particularly important point because at this moment much of the information required to complete the tables is not being collected by major industries. My second point pertains to the relation between regional and intraregional accounts. The authors tell us "all the accounts would provide data on totals not only for the entire urban region but for designated districts within the region as well." I am wondering whether the authors actually have in mind to provide current production and income accounts for subregions of a metropolitan area. Instead, what I would assume to be necessary is the development of the *associate accounts* for subregions. Even such an effort would pose major problems of aggregation and disaggregation, since it would have to be tied in to the over-all current production and income account.

May I also briefly raise an issue that greatly concerns me. Even today, and apparently it will be increasingly so in the future, urban areas are exhibiting very intricate intergovernmental fiscal relations. In addition, because of the great multiplicity of local governments and the mobility of resources, major spatial cost and benefit spillovers occur. They all have a bearing on equity and efficiency. Thus, urban areas would want to consider them in their decisions; and state and federal governments must likewise be aware of them. I would like to urge the authors to take one further look at their proposed regional government account with a view toward possibly increasing its ability to reflect these critical relations.

Altogether, Leven and Perloff convince us that further progress in developing the regional public-sector flow and stock accounts requires creative work along a number of major lines. For example, urban-government expenditures must be very carefully defined. To facilitate the making of public decisions, it might prove useful to define the cost of providing a public service as the opportunity cost, or the next best use of resources included in its provision. Opportunity cost is composed of direct and indirect cost, with the former including all costs for which money payments have been made and the latter involving the imputation of resource cost. Both direct and indirect costs can be further subdivided, depending on whether they are of current or capital nature. It is important to recognize that there are both capital expenditures that are incurred in a given year and annual debt-service charges. The latter, however, often do not properly reflect annual capital consumption, because of differences in the length of the debt-financing and useful-life periods, the handling of maintenance and its charges, and quality changes of the asset over time.

Likewise, it is important to clarify further the nature of government revenue and its measurement. Regional collection figures are grossly misleading, and yet spatial tax-incidence estimates are hard to come by.

Another important issue involves what should be included in the government account and what is the most appropriate government unit. It appears useful to reach an agreement on both issues in order to assure comparability of accounts in different parts of the country. Thus, the public-sector account might have three major components —government, social service agencies, and public utilities, i.e., services with user charges. Insofar as the appropriate government unit's permitting ready aggregation is concerned, it might be necessary to use municipality and special districts separately unless it becomes possible to allocate special district activities to municipalities by imputation. Large core cities and urban counties might have to be subdivided into neighborhoods.

In conclusion, I would like to reiterate my admiration for the contribution that I have been privileged to review. To use the homely phrase, that "the proof of the pudding is in the eating," I would like to urge others interested in the field of regional accounts to attempt to implement the proposals made by Leven and Perloff and in so doing, further refine the concepts and demonstrate their efficacy and applicability.

INDEX

Accounting systems, governmental, deficiencies in, 101–2, 104
Accounts:
　Definition, 107, 148–49
　Relating national, regional, and intraregional activities in, xi, xii
　See also National accounts; Regional accounts
Almindinger, V. V., 109n
Alonso, William, 158n
Amsterdam accounts, 57–58
Andrews, Richard B., 69n
Areal units. *See* Regions
Artle, Roland, 56, 88n

Becker, Gary, 52
Berliner, Joseph, 51n
Berman, Barbara R., 59, 88n, 89–90, 179n
Bloom, Clark, 51, 77
Blumen, Isadore, 162n
Bogue, Donald J., 153, 154
Bollens, John C., 57n
Borts, George H., 6n, 178n; comment of, 18–21
Brazer, Harvey E., comment of, 77–80
Brownlee, O. H., 63
Bureau of Labor Statistics data, 38, 173
Bureau of Old Age and Survivors Insurance data, 33, 154
Bureau of the Census:
　Current population survey, 172–173
　Post-enumeration survey, 161, 162
　See also Census data
Burkhead, Jesse, 87, 88, 90, 94, 102, 158: Paper by, xiv, 51–77; comment on, 77–85
　System of, data requirements, xiv–xv, 90–94; value of, 90, 94
Business Week, 40

Capital, role in regional accounts, 66–68, 73, 74, 75, 95–98, 184–85, 186, 198–200
Carroll, John, 64
Carrothers, Gerald A. P., 149n, 158n
Census data:
　Matching of, value in measuring mobility and migration, 162–63
　Uses of, 4, 6n, 7, 38, 89, 91–92, 99, 103–4, 118, 120, 166, 169, 171–73
Census systems:
　And registration systems, data gained through comparison, 161–62
　Measurement of human resources, 151–52, 153–54
Census tracts, value in data collection, 117, 128, 139
Chinitz, Benjamin, 59, 88n, 89n, 148, 149n, 158–59, 179n
Cities, evolution of, 53n, 136
Coale, Ansley J., 159n
Cochran, William G., 29n
Committee on Urban Economics, 128
Community, definition, 164
Commuters, interstate, estimating income, 34–38; comment, 46–49
Conference on Regional Accounts, first, xi, 175
Conference on Regional Accounts, second, xi–xii, xiii, 1, 107, 108
Converse, Muriel W., 80n
Correlation analysis, regional applications, 15–16
Cumberland, John H., 58n, 69n
Current population survey, 172–73
Current production and income account, 187–91, 198, 203; chart, 187
Current regional government account, value of, 68–69; table 72, 73, 75

215

Daicoff, Darwin W., 63n
Data:
    Collection and analysis, national programs proposed, 131–32
    Collection for human resources accounts, 151–57, 160–63; for manpower accounts, 171–74
    Government agencies supplying, 33, 38, 154, 173, 174. See also Census data; Unemployment-insurance data
    Intrametropolitan, program for organization and use, Niskanen paper, xv, 131–42; comment on, 143–46
    Regional centers for handling, 98–100, 132, 141–42, 146
    Requirements for manpower accounts, 166, 167, 171; for public finance account, xiv–xv, 87–105; for understanding regional growth, 205–7; for urban analysis and decision-making, 112, 114–15, 117, 121, 122, 125–27, 130, 131, 133–34, 142, 146, 176, 177–79, 181, 183
Data gaps, xv, 54, 88–90, 91–92, 95–98
Decision-making. See Policy-making
Delwart, Louis, 156n, 157, 178n
Department of Agriculture data, 174
Department of Commerce. See Office of Business Economics
deWolff, P., 57–58
Downs, Anthony, 55n
Dubos, René, 211
Duncombe, Bruce F., 5n, 8n
Dunn, Edgar S., Jr., 2n, 11n
Dunn, Halbert L., 154n

Econometric models, uses of, 182–83
Education expenditures, role in regional government account, 178, 200, 201, 201n, 212
Educational mobility, 156–57
Employment:
    Accounts for, 6, 9, 10, 20–21, 118–19, 122
    Population correlation, 10, 20–21
    Role in flow accounts, 186
    Role in human resources account, 194–96
    See also Manpower movements
Employment Security data. See Unemployment-insurance data
Evans, W. Duane, 191n

Federal government, role in regional government accounts, 61–62, 64
Federal Reserve Bank of Minneapolis, 40
Fein, Rashi, 147n
Ferguson, Charles E., comment of, 46–49
Finance. See Public finance
Fiscal planning, value of regional governments accounts in, 68
Fiscal relations, intergovernmental, role in regional planning, 213
Fisher, Joseph L., 158n
Fitch, Lyle C., comment of, 101–5
Flows:
    Accounts dealing with, regional analysis through, Henderson paper, xiii, 1–18, comment on, 18–23
    Data, inadequacy, 115
    Manpower, measurement of, 165–74
Flows and stocks:
    Applied to population, 149–50; modes of measurement, 151–54
    Relationships between, defined, 175n–76n
    Role in composition of social accounts, 115–16, 118, 128–30
    System of accounts dealing with: need for, xii, Perloff-Leven paper, xvii, xviii, 175–210; chart, 209; comment on, 210–14
Fox, Karl A., 109n; comment of, 80–85
Freedman, Deborah, 157n
Freedman, Ronald, 157n
From-to table for current production and income account, 190–91
From-to tables for manpower, xvii, 165–74
Functional relations, role in urban space model, 140, 142

Index

Geronymakis, Stylianos, 58n
Ginsberg, Eli, 147n
Gloversville accounts, 56
Goldstein, Sidney, 159n
Goodman, Leo A., 162n
Government, local, multiplicity of units, 64, 78, 213; conflicts of interest, 51–53, 78
Government sector:
  Decision-making, problems of, 70–71, 176–79
  Expenditures, autonomous and derived, distinguished, xiv, 70–71, 79–80
  History of treatment in regional accounting, 55–60
  Regional government accounts, Burkhead system, 60–71, 90–94; table, 72–77; Perloff-Leven system, 197–204, 212, 213, 214; chart, 199
  Role in current production and income account, 189
  Role in stock and flow accounts system, Perloff-Leven paper, xvii–xviii, 175–210; chart, 209; comment on, 210–14
  See also Public finance
Great Britain, regional accounts, 58–59

Haig, Robert M., 102n
Harris, Britton, 140–41, 149–50, 210; paper by, xvi, 107–27; comment on, 127–30
Hauser, Philip M., 153n, 161n
Health and well-being, measurement of, 53
Hearle, Edward F. R., 54n–55n, 141
Henderson, James M., paper by, xiii, 1–18; comment on, 18–23
Henry, Louis, 159n
Hirsch, Werner Z., 51n, 53, 57, 69, 98n, 131, 146, 154–55, 175n, 179n; introduction, xi–xviii; comment, 210–14
Hochwald, Werner, 51, 56, 57n, 59n, 63n, 70n, 88n, 141n, 149n, 152n, 154n, 156n, 157, 158n, 159n, 175n, 178n, 187n, 190n, 197n
Hoffenberg, Marvin, 191n

Hoover, Edgar M., 59, 88n, 89n, 112, 148, 149n, 158-59, 179n
Household sector. *See* Human resources
Housing, role in current production and income account, 189
Housing and Home Finance Agency, 132
Human resources accounting:
  Data collection for, 151–57, 160–63
  Importance of, xii
  Perloff-Leven account, 194–97, 198, 203n, 213; chart, 195
  Role in stock and flow accounts, 184–85, 186, 198, 200
  Schnore paper, xvi–xvii, 147–60; comment on, 160–64
  See also Manpower movements

Income, role in flow accounts, 186, 186n. *See also* Personal income
Income accounts:
  Concerned with policy, 44–46
  Current production and income account, 187–91, 198, 203; chart, 187
  Estimates of, preparing and assessing, Terry paper, xiii–xiv, 25–43; comment on, 43–49
  Interregional, 6–7, 9–10, 19–20
  National, as guide for regional, 25–26, 39, 44–45
Information. *See* Data
Input-output account, value of, xiii
Intrametropolitan data, organization and use, Niskanen paper, xv, 131–42; comment on, 143–46
Intraregional accounts:
  Need for integration with national and regional, xi, xii
  Perloff-Leven system, 204–5, 210, 213; chart, 205
Isard, Walter, 55, 58n, 69n, 164

Kalamazoo accounts, 56–57
Kansas City area, personal income in, 35–37, 47–49
Keynes, John Maynard, 45, 155
Kitagawa, Evelyn M., 153n, 161n
Koyan, Marvin, 162n

Labor force, role in human resources account, 194–97. *See also* Manpower
Labovitz, I. M., 63
Lampard, Eric E., 2n, 11n
Land use:
  And regional analysis, 69, 109, 110, 118, 119, 122, 185
  Basis of urban problems, 135
Leibenstein, Harvey, 159n
Leontief, W. W., 55, 170
Leven, Charles L., 41, 59, 63, 70, 88, 89, 149n, 187n, 190n, 197n; paper by, xvii–xviii, 175–210; comment on, 210–14
Linear programming, 108, 109
Local government, multiplicity of units, 64, 78; conflicts of interest, 51–53, 78
Local-government account, value, xii
Location:
  Importance in construction of social accounts, 111, 115, 116–18, 121–28
  Role in stock and flow accounts, 204, 205
  See also Migration; Social mobility; Space economy
Lowry, Ira S., comment of, 127–30

Mack, Ruth P., 183n; comment of, xiv, 43–46
Manpower movements as subject of regional accounts, Stolnitz paper, xvii, 165–74
Markets, external, effect on regional growth, 11–12
Mason, Raymond J., 141n
Massachusetts tax formula, 63, 78
Mattila, J. M., 16n
McCarthy, Philip J., 162n
Meier, Richard L., 149n
Metropolitan analysis:
  Accounts framework for, Harris paper, xvi, 107–27; comment on, 127–30
  Integrated system of accounts, Perloff-Leven paper, xvii–xviii, 175–210; comment on, 210–14
  Intrametropolitan data, organization and use, Niskanen paper, xv, 131–42; comment on, 143–46

Model of urban space economy, xv, 135–40; chart, 138; organization of data for, 140–42
Metropolitan planning, importance of welfare aspects, 110
Metropolitan region, feasibility as accounting unit, 159
Michigan tax study, 63
Microanalysis, limitation of, 182
Migration, data needed on, 152, 155–56; sources of, 162–63. *See also* Manpower movements
Mindlin, Albert, 146
Minnesota tax study, 63
Missouri, Kansas City area, personal income, 35–37, 47–49
Mobile (Ala.) accounts, 56
Mobility. *See* Social mobility
Models:
  Evolution and use of, 144–46
  Intrametropolitan, value in policy-making, 145–46
Moses, Leon N., xiii, 3n, 8n, 55
Mumford, Lewis, 53n
Musgrave, Richard A., 63n
Mushkin, Selma J., 94n, 147n
Muth, Richard F., 2n, 11n

National accounts:
  And regional accounts, xi, xii, 25–26, 39, 44–45, 179–80, 211
  Forms of, 148
Natural resources. *See* Non-human resources
Net in-area factor owner flow, defined, 41n–42n
Netzer, Dick, 51n, 110; paper by, xiv–xv, 87–100; comment on, 101–5
New York City accounts, 102–3
New York metropolitan region, xv, 59, 89–90, 95–98, 102, 104, 113
New York State, local-government activity, 64
Niskanen, William A., 107, 109; paper by, xv, 131–42; comment on, 143–46
Non-human resources:
  Account, 191–94, 213; chart, 193
  Role in stock and flow accounts, 184–85, 186, 198–200
Non-profit organizations, role in regional government accounts, 64–65

Northwestern University Transportation Center, xvi, 142

Office of Business Economics (OBE), personal income estimates, xiii, 25–40 *passim*
Opportunity cost, defined, 213–14
Orcutt, Guy, 131, 154n
Origin and destination studies, value, 114, 129, 130
Output, role in flow accounts, 4–6, 9, 186

Pappenfort, Donnell M., 164
Penn-Jersey Transportation Study, xv, 107, 108–10
Perloff, Harvey S., 2n, 11n, 51n, 54, 70, 99, 131, 151n, 152n, 155, 158, 178n, 197n; paper by, xvii–xviii, 175–210; comment on, 210–14
Personal income:
 Estimation, methods for, 40–49
 Estimation, OBE methods, xiii, 25–30; testing and appraisal, 30–40; tables, 31–32, 33
 Kansas City area, estimation method, 35–37; comment, 47–49
 State, defined, 26–27
 U.S. total for 1955, tables, 31–32, 33
 See also Income accounts
Pittsburgh regional economic study, 112, 140–41
Policy, regional, absence of orientation, 51–55; comment, 80–85
Policy-making:
 Long-term implications, 108, 110
 Problems of, 143–44, 176–79
 Role of regional accounts, xii, xviii, 70–71, 77–78, 79, 158–59; government, 65–69, 79, 81–85; income, 44–46; locational, 121–23; stock-flow, 176, 186, 200, 210
 Value of models, 135–36, 144–46
 Value of organized system of data, 133–35
Population:
 Employment correlation, 10, 20–21
 Migration and mobility, accounts on, 7–8, 20–21, 22–23; data needed, 155–57

Role in economic analysis, 147; in human resources account, 196–97; in metropolitan accounts, 118, 122; in regional government account, 200, 201; in urban decision-making, 177–78
 See also Human resources
Position rents, use in model-building, 109, 139–40
Post-enumeration survey, 161, 162
President's Committee to Appraise Employment and Unemployment Statistics, 172, 173
Prest, A. R., 63n
Production and income account, current, 187–91, 198, 203; chart, 187
Property, role in urban decision-making, 177–78
Proxy allocators and extrapolators, explained, 29
Public finance and regional accounts, 186, 197–204, 213, 214; Burkhead paper and comment, xiv, 51–80; data requirements, Netzer paper and comment, 87–105
Public sector. *See* Government sector
Public services, role in regional government account, 200, 201–3
Puerto Rico, accounting system, revision, 104–5

RAND Corp., xvi, 54n–55n, 109, 142
Regional accounts:
 And national accounts, xi, xii, 25–26, 39, 44–45, 179–80, 211
 Capital budget for New York metropolitan region, 95–98
 Core and subsidiary, xii–xiii
 Data requirements. *See* Data
 Definition of "accounts," 107, 148–49
 Functions of, 175
 Government: Burkhead system, 65–71, 79, 90–94; table, 72–77; Perloff-Leven system, 197–204, 212, 213, 214; chart, 199
 Human resources. *See* Human resources accounting
 Income. *See* Income accounts
 Manpower movements, xvii, 167–74
 Metropolitan. *See* Metropolitan analysis

Public finance, xiv, 51–80; data requirements for, xiv–xv, 87–105
Public sector, history of treatment, 55–60
Role in policy-making. *See* Policy-making
Role of taxes in, 62–64, 68, 78–79, 189–90, 203–4
Social. *See* Social accounts
System based on interregional flows, 3–11, 18–23
System for regional projection and explanation, 13–18, 19–21
System relating stocks and flows, xvii–xviii, 175–214; chart, 209
Regional analysis:
Absence of policy orientation, 51–55; comment, 80–85
Comparisons, regional-national, as means of, xii, 2–3, 11–12
Data requirements, *See* Data
Goals of, 78
Role of land use, 69, 109, 110, 118, 119, 122, 185
See also Regional accounts
Regional data centers, 98–100, 132, 141–42, 146
Regional growth and change, role of regional accounts in understanding, xi, xviii, 175, 178, 179, 180–81, 183–84, 205–7
Regional Plan Association, 95, 96
Regions, problem of definition. 157–59, 163–64, 167–68
Registration systems:
And census systems, data gained through comparison, 161–62
Continuous, question of, xvii, 153–54, 155, 160, 171
Measurement of human resources, 152–54, 159n
Regression analysis, regional applications, 15–17
Reiner, Thomas A., 164
Resources. *See* Human resources; Nonhuman resources
Rivlin, Alice M., 147n
Rodd, R. Stephen, 6n
Rodwin, Lloyd, 69n
Ruggles, Nancy D., 148n, 157–58
Ruggles, Richard, 148n, 157–58

Sacks, Seymour, 64
St. Louis accounts, 57, 69
Sales Management, 40
Sandee, J., 81
Schaller, Howard G., 69n, 98n
Schnore, Leo F., paper by, xvi–xvii, 147–60; comment on, 160–64
School construction, problem of decision-making on, 178
Schultz, Theodore W., 147n
Shoup, Carl S., 102n
Sioux City accounts, 88–89
Situs problem, 47–49
Sjaastad, Larry A., 7n
Smith, Harold T,. 57
SMSA's. *See* Standard Metropolitan Statistical Areas
Social accounts:
Categories, interrelation of, 117–18, 119–21
Importance of location in construction of, 111, 115, 116–18, 121–28
Kinds needed, 118–19, 121–22
Two varieties of, 149
See also Human resources accounting; Metropolitan analysis
Social costs of government and private activity, 52, 53
Social mobility:
Concept applied to social accounting, 150
Data on, 152, 156–57, 162–63
Social Security Administration data, 173
Social-security numbers, value in identification, 162, 163
Sonenblum, Sidney, 56, 57n, 88n, 156n, 157, 178n; comment of, 21–23
Space economy, urban, model of, xv, 135–40; chart, 138; organization of data for, 140–42
Space requirements. *See* Land use
Standard Metropolitan Statistical Areas, role in regional analysis, 2, 3, 64
State governments, role in regional government accounts, 62, 64
Stein, Jerome L. 178n
Stockholm accounts, 56
Stocks and flows. *See* Flows and stocks

Index

Stolnitz, George J., paper by, xvii, 165–74
Stone-Deane accounts for Great Britain, 58–59
Striner, Herbert E., 56, 57n, 88n
Suits, Daniel B., 80n
Survey of Current Business, personal income estimates. *See* Office of Business Economics
Sweden, registration system, xvii, 153–54

Taxes, role in regional accounts, 62–64, 68, 78–79, 94, 189–90, 203–4
Tenner, Irving, 101
Terry, Edwin F., paper by, xiii–xiv, 25–43; comment on, 43–49
Theil, H., 81
Thomas, Dorothy S., 153
Thompson, W. R., 16n
Tiebout, Charles M., 190
Tinbergen, Jan, model of national economy, 81–85, 109
Trade:
In Upper Midwest, account system, 14–15
Interregional accounts, 4–6, 8–9, 10, 18–23
Theory of international, value in study of interregional, 2–3, 18
See also Flows

Transportation:
Accounts for, 118, 119, 122, 208, 210
Penn-Jersey study, xv, 107, 108–10
Studies of, value, 114, 115, 127, 129

Unemployment-insurance data, value of, 6, 6n, 33, 34, 37–38, 47, 118
Upper Midwest Economic Study, 5, 8, 13, 18–20
Urban. *See* Metropolitan
Use, measurement in interregional trade accounts, 4–5; demand coefficients, 9–10

Van Eijk, C. J., 81
Venekamp, P. E., 57–58
Vernon, Raymond, 95, 112, 113

Weisbrod, Burton A., 184n
Welfare aspects of metropolitan planning, 110
Whitney, Vincent Heath, 159n
Wingo, Lowdon, Jr., xvi, 134; comment of, 143–46
Winkler, Wilhelm, 159n
Winsborough, Hal H., xvii; comment of, 160–64
Wolfle, Dael, 147n

HC
106.5
C6734
1962a